Lecture Notes in Computer Science   8361

Commenced Publication in 1973
Founding and Former Series Editors:
Gerhard Goos, Juris Hartmanis, and Jan van Leeuwen

For further volumes:
http://www.springer.com/series/7412

Marius Erdt · Marius George Linguraru
Cristina Oyarzun Laura · Raj Shekhar
Stefan Wesarg · Miguel Angel González Ballester
Klaus Drechsler (Eds.)

Clinical Image-Based Procedures

Translational Research in Medical Imaging

Second International Workshop, CLIP 2013
Held in Conjunction with MICCAI 2013
Nagoya, Japan, September 22, 2013
Revised Selected Papers

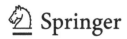 Springer

Editors
Marius Erdt
Fraunhofer IDM@NTU
Singapore
Singapore

Marius George Linguraru
Raj Shekhar
Children's National Medical Center
Washington, DC
USA

Cristina Oyarzun Laura
Stefan Wesarg
Klaus Drechsler
Fraunhofer IGD
Darmstadt
Germany

Miguel Angel González Ballester
ICREA – Universitat Pompeu Fabra
Barcelona
Spain

ISSN 0302-9743　　　　ISSN 1611-3349　(electronic)
ISBN 978-3-319-05665-4　　ISBN 978-3-319-05666-1　(eBook)
DOI 10.1007/978-3-319-05666-1
Springer Cham Heidelberg New York Dordrecht London

Library of Congress Control Number: 2014934687

LNCS Sublibrary: SL6 – Image Processing, Computer Vision, Pattern Recognition, and Graphics

Printed on acid-free paper

Springer is part of Springer Science+Business Media (www.springer.com)

Preface

On September 22, 2013, the Second International Workshop on Clinical Image-based Procedures: Translational Research in Medical Imaging (CLIP 2013) was held in Nagoya, Japan, in conjunction with the 16th International Conference on Medical Image Computing and Computer-Assisted Intervention (MICCAI). This successful workshop was a productive and exciting forum for the discussion and dissemination of clinically tested, state-of-the-art methods for image-based planning, monitoring, and evaluation of medical procedures.

Over the past few years, there has been considerable and growing interest in the development and evaluation of new translational image-based procedures in the modern hospital. For a decade or more, a proliferation of meetings dedicated to medical image computing has created a need for greater study and scrutiny of the clinical application and validation of such methods. New attention and new strategies are essential to ensure a smooth and effective translation of computational image-based techniques into the clinic. For these reasons, the major focus of CLIP 2013 was on translational research filling the gaps between basic science and clinical applications.

Members of the medical imaging community were encouraged to submit work centered on specific clinical applications, including techniques and procedures based on comprehensive clinical image data. The event brought together some 50 world-class researchers and clinicians who presented ways to strengthen links between computer scientists and engineers as well as surgeons, interventional radiologists, and radiation oncologists.

Thus, CLIP 2013 was a successful forum for the dissemination of emerging image-based clinical techniques. Specific topics included pre-interventional image segmentation and classification (to support diagnosis and clinical decision making), interventional and surgical planning and analysis of dynamic images, and evaluation, visualization, and correction techniques for image-based procedures. Clinical applications covered orthopedics, the skull and the brain, blood vessels, abdominal organs, endoscopic interventions, and cancer in adults and children. The presentations and discussions around the meeting emphasized current challenges and emerging techniques in image-based procedures, strategies for clinical translation of image-based techniques, the role of computational anatomy and image analysis for surgical planning and interventions, and the contribution of medical image analysis to open and minimally invasive surgery. During two keynote sessions, clinical highlights were presented and discussed by Prof. Makoto Hashizume, MD PhD, from Kyushu University School of Medicine in Japan (minimally invasive robotic surgery), and Prof. Nobuhiko Sugano, MD PhD, from Osaka University Graduate School of Medicine, Japan (computer-assisted orthopedic surgery). We are grateful to our keynote speakers for their compelling presentations. We would also like to acknowledge the European

Commission research project HEAR-EU (grant number HEALTH-F2-2012-304857) for providing support for the participation of the keynote speakers.

In response to the call for papers, 26 original manuscripts were submitted for presentation at CLIP 2013. Each of the manuscripts underwent a meticulous double-blind peer review by a minimum of two members of the Program Committee, all of them prestigious experts in the field of medical image analysis and clinical translations of technology. Finally, 50 % of the manuscripts (i.e., 13 papers) were accepted for oral presentation at the workshop, and an additional six papers were accepted for poster presentation combined with a short oral summary of their work, bringing the overall acceptance rate to 73 %. The six papers with the highest review score were nominated to be considered as best papers. The three best papers were chosen by votes cast by workshop participants who had attended all six presentations of the nominated papers (excluding workshop organizers). As a result, three awards were presented. First place went to Xin Kang, Jihun Oh, Emmanuel Wilson, Timothy Kane, Craig Peters, and Raj Shekhar from Children's National Medical Center in Washington, DC, USA for their work on a novel stereoscopic augmented reality system for laparoscopic surgery. Second place was presented to Adrian Schneider, Christian Baumberger, Mathias Griessen, Simon Pezold, Jörg Beinemann, Philipp Jürgens, and Philippe C. Cattin from Universität Basel, Switzerland, for their work on landmark-based surgical navigation. Third place was conferred on Carles Sánchez, Jorge Bernal, F. Javier Sánchez, and Debora Gil from Universitat Autónoma de Barcelona in Spain for their advancements regarding lumen center detection in gastrointestinal and respiratory endoscopy. We would like to congratulate warmly all the prize winners for their outstanding work and exciting presentations and thank our sponsors, EXOCAD and MedCom, for their support.

We would like to acknowledge the invaluable contributions of our entire Program Committee without whose assistance CLIP2013 would not have been as successful and stimulating. Our thanks also go to all the authors in this volume for the high quality of their work and their commitment of time and effort. Finally, we are grateful to the MICCAI organizers, and particularly Hongen Liao, Akinobu Shimizu, Pierre Jannin, and Simon Warfield for supporting the organization of CLIP 2013.

December 2013

Miguel A. González Ballester
Klaus Drechsler
Marius Erdt
Marius George Linguraru
Cristina Oyarzun Laura
Raj Shekhar
Stefan Wesarg

Organization

Organizing Committee

Klaus Drechsler   Fraunhofer IGD, Germany
Marius Erdt   Fraunhofer IDM@NTU, Singapore
Miguel A. González Ballester   ICREA – Universitat Pompeu Fabra Alma IT Systems, Spain
Marius George Linguraru   Children's National Medical Center, USA
Cristina Oyarzun Laura   Fraunhofer IGD, Germany
Raj Shekhar   Children's National Medical Center, USA
Stefan Wesarg   Fraunhofer IGD, Germany

Program Committee

Mario Ceresa   Alma IT Systems, Spain
Juan Cerrolaza   Children's National Medical Center, USA
Yufei Chen   Tongji University, China
Jan Egger   University of Marburg, Germany
Wissam El Hakimi   Technische Universität Darmstadt, Germany
Gloria Fernández Esparrach   Hospital Clinic Barcelona, Spain
Moti Freimann   Harvard Medical School, USA
Enrico Grisan   University of Padova, Italy
Tobias Heimann   Siemens, Germany
Xin Kang   Children's National Medical Center, USA
Matthias Keil   Fraunhofer IGD, Germany
Michael Kelm   Siemens Corporate Research, Germany
Matthias Kirschner   Technische Universität Darmstadt, Germany
Yoshitaka Masutani   Tokyo University, Japan
Jihun Oh   Children's National Medical Center, USA
Danielle Pace   Kitware Inc., USA
Mauricio Reyes   University of Bern, Switzerland
Akinobu Shimizu   Tokyo University of Agriculture and Technology, Japan
Ronald M. Summers   National Institutes of Health, USA
Kenji Suzuki   University of Chicago, USA
Zeike Taylor   University of Sheffield, UK
Diana Wald   German Cancer Research Center, Germany
Thomas Wittenberg   Fraunhofer IIS, Germany

Qian Zhao   Children's National Medical Center, USA
Ziv Yaniv   Children's National Medical Center, USA
Stephan Zidowitz   Fraunhofer Mevis, Germany

Sponsoring Institutions

exocad GmbH, Germany
MedCom GmbH, Germany

Contents

Statistical Analysis of Relative Pose of the Thalamus in Preterm Neonates

Yi Lao[1,2(✉)], Jie Shi[4], Yalin Wang[4], Rafeal Ceschin[5], Darryl Hwang[2],
M.D. Nelson[1], Ashok Panigrahy[5], and Natasha Leporé[1,2,3]

[1] Department of Radiology, Children's Hospital Los Angeles, Los Angeles, CA, USA
yilao1987@gmail.com
[2] Department of Biomedical Engineering, University of Southern California,
Los Angeles, CA, USA
[3] Department of Radiology, University of Southern California, Los Angeles, CA, USA
[4] School of Computing, Informatics, and Decision Systems Engineering,
Arizona State University, Tempe, AZ, USA
[5] Department of Radiology, Children's Hospital of Pittsburgh UPMC,
Pittsburgh, PA, USA

Abstract. Preterm neonates are at higher risk of neurocognitive and neurosensory abnormalities. While numerous studies have looked at the effect of prematurity on brain anatomy, none to date have attempted to understand the relative pose of subcortical structures and to assess its potential as a biomarker of abnormal growth. Here, we perform the first relative pose analysis on a point distribution model (PDM) of the thalamus between 17 preterm and 19 term-born healthy neonates. Initially, linear registration and constrained harmonic registration were computed to remove the irrelevant global pose information and obtain correspondence in vertices. All the parameters for the relative pose were then obtained through similarity transformation. Subsequently, all the pose parameters (scale, rotation and translation) were projected into a log-Euclidean space, where univariate and multivariate statistics were performed. Our method detected relative pose differences in the preterm birth for the left thalamus. Our results suggest that relative pose in subcortical structures is a useful indicator of brain injury, particularly along the anterior surface and the posterior surface. Our study supports the concept that there are regional thalamic asymmetries in the preterm that may be related to subtle white matter injury, have prognostic significance, or be related to preterm birth itself.

1 Introduction

Being born prematurely is a risk factor to lifelong neurocognitive and neurosensory deficits (see e.g. [8,13]). Abnormalities have been detected in several areas of the brain of premature newborns, including subcortical structures such as the thalamus [3,12]. The thalamus is a 'switch board' structure in the brain which starts its formation as early as the 15th gestational week [5]. As a result, it is likely a sensitive indicator of prematurity, and this structure has been the focus of

M. Erdt et al. (Eds.): CLIP 2013, LNCS 8361, pp. 1–9, 2014.
DOI: 10.1007/978-3-319-05666-1_1, © Springer International Publishing Switzerland 2014

several brain anatomy studies associated with preterm birth. Reduced thalamic volumes associated with preterm birth have been documented through several MRI studies [12]. In particular, [14] detected statistically significant morphological changes in the left thalamus using multivariate tensor-based morphometry (mTBM).

While maturity is a continuous process that spans the first few years of life, the first several months after birth are especially critical since the growth exhibits an outward expanding trend with evident subcortical structure changes, in terms of size, shape and relative pose within the brain. Complementary to size and shape analysis, the relative pose of subcortical structures may help to indicate the abnormal growth of the brain. This information is especially important in depicting the developing or degeneration patterns of the brain, when shifts of pose in different subcortical structures are more likely to happen. In brain degeneration studies, [1] successfully detected brain atrophy associated pose changes in Alzheimer's disease. However, to our knowledge, few or no pose information is included in prematurity studies and relative pose has not yet been studies in relation to brain development. Here, we use similarity transformations to align the thalamus of each subject, and perform univariate as well as multivariate analyses on so-generated pose parameters, thus investigating the effect of prematurity on the relative pose between preterm and term-born neonates at term-equivalent age. We tested the hypothesis that we may detect regional differences in thalamic relative pose in preterms with no visible injury compared to term controls.

There are two major contributions in this paper. First, we developed a novel pose analysis system that integrates various brain surface processing techniques including parametrization and constrained harmonic registration and reports the subtle pose changes on subcortical structures. The obtained pose information is complementary to subcortical surface shape analyses, and the combined shape and pose results form a complete subcortical morphometry system. Secondly, we applied the system to study prematurity. Our preliminary results indicate that the pose analysis information is consistent with prior discoveries, so our work provides a novel tool for brain research in neonates.

2   Subjects and Methodology

2.1   Neonatal Data

T1-weighted MRI scans consisting of 17 preterm neonates (gestational ages 25-36 weeks, 41.12 ± 5.08 weeks at scan time) and 19 term born infants (gestational ages 37–40 weeks, 45.51 ± 5.40 weeks at scan time) were acquired using dedicated neonatal head coils on 1.5T GE scanners, with coronal 3D spoiled gradient echo (SPGR) sequence. All the subjects in our datasets were classified into a preterm group and term group by 2 neonatal neuroradiologists. Preterm neonates included in this study were less than 37 gestational weeks at birth, and without visible injuries on MR scans. Subjects with abnormal MR scans were excluded in our datasets.

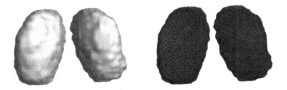

Fig. 1. 3D surface model of the left and the right thalamus and their corresponding mesh grids from one subject.

2.2   Point Distribution Model

All the T1-weighted MRI scans were first registered to a same template space through linear registration. Alignment quality was validated by superimposing images from differenct subjects on top of each other. Irrelevant global pose difference induced by different locations and orientations during scans was factored out in this step. The thalami were then manually traced on linear registered T1 images by an experienced pediatric neuroradiologist using Insight Toolkit's SNAP program [16]. The intra-rater percentage overlap were 0.93 for the thalamus, in four participants at two subsequent times (two preterm and two term born participants). Based on binary segmentations, 3D surface representations of the thalamus were constructed and mesh grids were built on the surfaces by computing surface conformal parameterizations with holomorphic 1-forms, using our in-house conformal mapping program. Figure 1 shows an example of a reconstructed surface, and corresponding mesh grids on a thalamus. One-to-one correspondence between vertices were obtained through a constrained harmonic registration algorithm [15].

2.3   Similarity Transformation

For each thalamus, the relative pose was obtained by a full Procrustes fit of a template shape to the PDM. The template shape was selected as the mean shape that minimized the Procrustes distances, and it was computed iteratively [11]. Full Procrustes alignment means that the similarity transformation is estimated in terms of a uniform scale, a rotation and a translation in x, y and z directions [4]. To be more specific, here, the transformations were centered according to the center of mass of the mean shape. The transformation rule of Procrustes alignment is defined as [1], $T\langle X \rangle = (sRX, d)$, where s is the scalar scaling factor, R is a 3×3 rotation matrix and d is the translation vector $(x, y, z)^T$. To form a Lie group with matrix multiplication, the matrix representation of the Procrustes transformation can be written as [2]:

$$T = \begin{pmatrix} sRX & d \\ 0^T & 1 \end{pmatrix} \qquad (1)$$

To simplify computations, all the parameters of the transformations were projected onto a log-Euclidean space - the tangent plane at the origin of the transformation group manifold. Because these similarity transformations form a Lie group, projections can be computed as matrix logarithms and exponentials as explained in [2].

In group studies, it is intuitive to define a mean. Similar to Euclidean space, here the mean in Lie group was defined as the point which minimized the squared distance [6], and the mean pose can be calculated iteratively as follow [1,10]:

$$m_{k+1} = m_k exp(\frac{1}{n}\sum_{i=1}^{n} log(m_k^{-1}T_i)).\qquad(2)$$

After the subtraction of the mean from each subject's individual pose, specifically using $v_i = log(m^{-1}T_i)$, each subject is left with a residual pose. Statistics are computed on the residual pose which consists of 7 parameters: 1 scale scalar, 3 rotation scalars and 3 translation scalars.

2.4 Statistical Analysis

Although the mean and distribution of age was roughly matched between preterm and term groups, subjects were scanned over an age range of 36–57 postconception weeks. This variation of age is not negligible, especially for neonates, whose

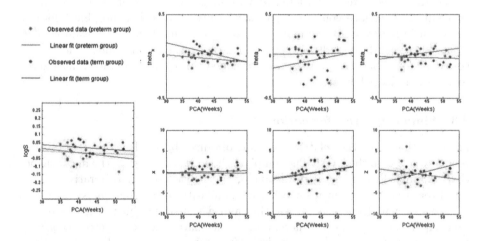

Fig. 2. Distribution of 7 pose parameters in log-Euclidean space for the left thalamus: logS, $(\theta_x, \theta_y, \theta_z)$, (x, y, z). Stars in the figure represent observed data from Procrustes alignment, while lines represent their corresponding linear regressions. In all the figures above, data from preterm group are marked in red, and data from term group are marked in blue. Note that logS is approximately constant with post-conception age, indicating that the thalamus volume is near constant in that age range. However, a downward slope is seen in the preterm group. When very preterm subjects are removed from the sample (postconception age at birth <31 weeks), the linear regression (shown in a cyan) for preterm subjects normalizes to a flat line, indicating a similar behavior to the term born subjects (Color figure online).

brains change rapidly with age. The distributions of 7 pose parameters are shown in Fig. 2; to save the space, only the data from the left thalamus are presented. The growth of the thalamus in neonates in terms of the volumetry and outgoing trajectory is approximately linear, thus we used linear regression to factor out the influence of age. Subsequent statistical analyses were performed on age-covariated data. It is important to note that although log S is approximately steady with age in the term group, the tread in the preterm group is saliently decreased. This is due to the existence of extremely preterm subjects (born 25–31 gestational weeks). A linear regression line of preterm data excluding the extremely preterm cases is also shown in the same panel in cyan color in Fig. 3. The line is close to constant as in the term born case.

Statistical comparisons between the two groups were performed via two methods: univariate t-test for logS, $||logR||$, $||logd||$, $\theta_x,\theta_y,\theta_z$, x, y, z; Multivariate

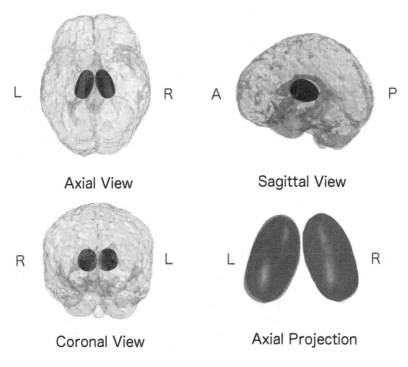

| | Axial View | | Sagittal View | |
| L | | R   A | | P |

| | Coronal View | | Axial Projection | |
| R | | L   L | | R |

Fig. 3. 3D visualization of the pose of mean shapes averaged from preterm group (Red) and term group (Blue). The relative position of thalamus are presented in a transparent head, shown in Axial, Sagittal and Coronal views. A close look of the Axial view is shown in the bottom right corner: areas where the mean shapes of two groups overlaid appear in purple. Note the borders of these two structures: shift of pose is evident on the left thalamus, while less visible variants appear on the right thalamus. In addition, there appears to be more shifting of the anterior and posterior ends of the thalamus which co-localize to the pulvinar (posterior) and the medial dorsal and anterior nucleus (anterior) (Color figure online).

Hotelling's T^2-test, which is a multivariate generalization of the t-test, for 3 rotation parameters $(\theta_x, \theta_y, \theta_z)$, 3 translation parameters (x, y, z), a combination of $logS$, $||logR||$, and $||logd||$, as well as a combination of all 7 parameters.

Considering the limited size of our dataset (36 subjects), a permutation test [9] was performed to avoid the normal distribution assumption. To do this, we randomly permuted the labels of our subjects (preterm vs. term neonates), and generated t-values (for t-test) or F-values (for T^2-test) for comparison. We used 10000 permutations for each of the parameters to assemble a null distribution of nonparametric estimation for t- or F-values.

3   Results

All the p-values from previously described tests are presented in Table 1. As we can see from the table, for the left thalamus, pose parameters representing scale and rotation show a significant difference between the preterm and term groups, while no difference can be seen in translation parameters. It is also important to note that, apart from the difference detected in individual parameters, a combination of all 7 parameters also detected significant differences between the two groups in the left thalamus, indicating a possibility of using multivariate analysis of all pose parameters as the discriminant between the two populations. For the right thalamus, neither the individual or combination of parameters detected any changes.

These results are better visualized in Fig. 3, where mean shapes of preterm (represented in red) vs. term (represented in blue) groups are overlaid in their corresponding mean pose. The left thalamus of the preterm group showed a smaller size as well as an inward tendency compared to the term group, which is consistent with the differences found in scale and rotation parameters. Compared

Table 1. P-value of statistical analyses on pose parameters: 13 sets of parameters characterizing relative pose of left thalamus (LTha) and right thalamus (RTha) are investigated here using univariate and multivariate analyses. Parameters are categorized as logS, $||logR||$, $||logd||$, $\theta_x, \theta_y, \theta_z$, x, y, and z for univariate tests, and as $(\theta_x, \theta_y, \theta_z)$, (x, y, z), $(logS, ||logR||, ||logd||)$, and a combination of 7 parameters for multivariate tests. All the p-values are obtained after permutation testing. Significant p-values ($p < 0.05$) are highlighted in light cyan, while p-values that are interestingly low but failed to reach significance are highlighted in light grey (Color table online).

	LTha	RTha		LTha	RTha
$logS$	2.27e-02	3.43e-01	$||logR||$	5.75e-01	5.73e-01
θ_x	5.60e-03	6.49e-01	$||logd||$	8.88e-01	4.00e-01
θ_y	1.94e-01	9.21e-01	$(\theta_x, \theta_y, \theta_z)$	9.80e-03	7.14e-01
θ_z	5.29e-02	2.61e-01	(x, y, z)	8.41e-01	8.23e-01
x	4.97e-01	8.85e-01	$(logS, ||logR||, ||logd||)$	1.76e-01	4.67e-01
y	8.40e-01	4.85e-01	$All 7 paras$	2.05e-02	9.17e-01
z	6.35e-01	4.90e-01			

to the obvious differences in size and shape, the shift of position of the left thalamus in these two groups are less evident, thus further validating the less significant result from translation parameters. As for the right thalamus, we can see mean shapes from these 2 groups are mostly overlapped, only a slight size difference is shown in Fig. 3. These are also consistent with the relatively high p-value found in the scale, rotation and translation parameters.

4   Discussion

Here, we introduced a relative pose analysis into the prematurity associated brain anatomy analyses. Our pose computation successfully detected differences in the left thalamus in preterm neonates, while no difference in terms of relative pose was detected on the right thalamus between preterm and term neonates. The two thalami in the brain are not exactly symmetric in terms of functions, and hemispheric asymmetries in the thalamus have been well-documented via animal studies [7]. Our results provide additional information about the developing patterns of the two thalami.

Before our study, a reduction in thalamic volume in preterm infants compared to term-born controls was shown by manual volumetry study [12]. The reductions are consistent with the significant differences in the scale parameter we found here. However, in the volumetry study, the left and right thalami are treated as a whole, thus failing to localize the differences within the two thalami. A recent surface morphometry study has found significant regional differences on the surface of the left thalamus [14], while fewer surface changes are detected in the right thalamus. Complementary to these results, the pose information we found in our study further confirms that the left thalamus may be more vulnerable to prematurity. In addition, the relative pose information also revealed regional differences which co-localize to known nuclear subdivision in the thalamus (i.e. pulvinar and medial dorsal nucleus) which have been previously shown to be abnormal in preterm neonates relative to term controls. Here, we demonstrate for the first time that relative pose can help with delineating regional changes of the preterm thalamus, with respect to the anterior and posterior poles of the left thalamus.

Moreover, in very preterm subjects, the scale parameter is reduced with postconception age. This supports the existence of regional vulnerability of the preterm thalamus, in the setting of no visible white matter injury. Our data suggest that even when there are global subtle volumetric difference related to the degree of prematurity, relative pose (likely in combination with surface TBM) may assist with delineating regional thalamic changes.

Our work proposes a complete set of relative pose statistics based on more accurate subcortical structure registrations: Firstly, our study used an accurate mesh representation consisting of 15,000 surface points, and point correspondences were obtained by a constrained harmonic registration, which outperforms traditional algorithms in matching the large differences between neonatal brain volumes, thus yielding higher accuracy. Secondly, post statistics are performed using both univariate and multivariate analyses on different combinations of pose parameters and their norms, to find the most sensitive statistical marker for prematurity associated differences. Finally, this is the first time that the trend of pose parameters vs. PCA has been computed. There is little research on pose in brain structure in general, and none in neonates. Our work may lead to new biomarkers for prematurity.

There are several possible limitations in this study: (1) the effect of age was removed using linear regression, however, for some of our parameters such as θ_y and Ty, Tz (Fig. 2), the linear model may not best describe the age-dependent changes. Therefore, a more dedicated age-covariant model is needed in future studies. (2) Our study is limited to a relatively small number of subjects. We plan to increase our sample size in the future to confirm results found here, and correlating our findings with neurodevelopmental outcomes. In addition, we plan to examine the relative pose of different subcortical structures (i.e. putamen, hippocampus and thalamus) in relation to reach other in preterm neonates relative to term controls, which may shed light on the global effects of prematurity on grey matter structures.

References

1. Bossa, M., et al.: Statistical analysis of relative pose information of subcortical nuclei: application on ADNI data. Neuroimage **55**(3), 999–1008 (2011)
2. Bossa, M.N., et al.: Statistical model of similarity transformations: building a multi-object pose model of brain structures. In: IEEE Computer Society Workshop on Mathematical Methods in Biomedical Image Analysis, p. 59 (2006)
3. Counsell, S.J., et al.: Thalamo-cortical connectivity in children born preterm mapped using probabilistic magnetic resonance tractography. Neuroimage **34**(3), 896–904 (2007)
4. Dryden, I., et al.: Statistical Analysis of Shape. Wiley, New York (1998)
5. Glenn, O.A.: Normal development of the fetal brain by MRI. Semin. Perinatol. **33**, 208–219 (2009). (Elsevier)
6. Karcher, H.: Riemannian center of mass and mollifier smoothing. Commun. Pure Appl. Math. **30**(5), 509–541 (1977)
7. King, C., et al.: Thalamic asymmetry is related to acoustic signal complexity. Neurosci. Lett. **267**(2), 89–92 (1999)
8. Marlow, N., et al.: Neurologic and developmental disability at six years of age after extremely preterm birth. N. Engl. J. Med. **352**(1), 9–19 (2005)
9. Nichols, T.E., et al.: Nonparametric permutation tests for functional neuroimaging: a primer with examples. Hum. Brain Mapp. **15**(1), 1–25 (2001)
10. Pennec, X., et al.: A Riemannian framework for tensor computing. Int. J. Comput. Vision **66**(1), 41–66 (2006)
11. Ross, A.: Procrustes analysis. Course report, Department of Computer Science and Engineering, University of South Carolina (2004)
12. Srinivasan, L., et al.: Quantification of deep gray matter in preterm infants at term-equivalent age using manual volumetry of 3-tesla magnetic resonance images. Pediatrics **119**(4), 759–765 (2007)

13. Vohr, B.R., et al.: Neurodevelopmental and functional outcomes of extremely low birth weight infants in the national institute of child health and human development neonatal research network, 1993–1994. Pediatrics **105**(6), 1216–1226 (2000)
14. Wang, Y., et al.: Surface morphometry of subcortical structures in premature neonates. Proc. Intl. Soc. Mag. Reson. Med. **19**, 2585 (2011)
15. Wang, Y., et al.: Surface-based TBM boosts power to detect disease effects on the brain: an N=804 ADNI study. Neuroimage **56**(4), 1993–2010 (2011)
16. Zhang, H., et al.: Deformable registration of diffusion tensor MR images with explicit orientation optimization. Med. Image Anal. **10**(5), 764–785 (2006)

Forming the Interface Between Doctor and Designing Engineer

Christine Schoene$^{(\boxtimes)}$, Philipp Sembdner, Stefan Holzhausen,
and Ralph Stelzer

Faculty of Mechanical Science and Engineering,
Technische Universitaet Dresden, Dresden, Germany
{Christine.Schoene, Philipp.Sembdner,
Stefan.Holzhausen, Ralph.Stelzer}@tu-dresden.de

Abstract. In the medical domain, the use of biocompatible materials, such as titanium or titanium alloys is essential to produce individual implants. As a result of this development, it is now possible to generate new patient-specific geometries fitted to the contour. This paper elucidates the process chain to derive individual design variants and to produce patient-specific bone replacement implants for the lower jaw-bone regions by using innovative reverse engineering and manufacturing methods based on CT-data. For this interdisciplinary project, technical scientists, medical scientists at the university hospital and engineers from a product development firm work together.

Keywords: Process chain · Planning implants · CT-data

1 Purpose

As a result of ongoing globalisation, the greatly expanding market for medical implants made of biocompatible high-performance materials is under ever-increasing pressure from competitors. In this context, the reconstruction of bone defects, in particular in the oral, jaw and facial region, by means of osteosynthetic plates is regarded as a great challenge. Here, special advantages may accrue to a new implant design whose contour and stiffness are tailored to specific geometric and elastic conditions, since in this way it is possible to reduce complications during ingrowth. One objective of the research project is aimed at the development of a process chain that extends all the way from CT layer images of a diseased patient up to the manufacturing of individual bone substitute implants for the patient while taking into consideration a Rapid Manufacturing technique [1–3].

In this context, manufacturing of individualized medical products supported by customized software solutions is becoming more and more important. However, these software tools must be designed so that they are easy to handle and understand. It is not feasible to assume that the surgeon will devote much time to becoming familiar with the software. Also a wide variety of functions may be a liability, in that it is often one reason for the rejection of a product.

M. Erdt et al. (Eds.): CLIP 2013, LNCS 8361, pp. 10–14, 2014.
DOI: 10.1007/978-3-319-05666-1_2, © Springer International Publishing Switzerland 2014

Individualised medical products are created in a series of carefully synchronised and mutually interlocking process steps. In this process, doctors, designing engineers and production planners work together in an interdisciplinary team. Consequently, project work within the process chain has to be supported and optimised through customised software tools in order to create an immediate interface for communication and data exchange.

One example that illustrates the need for such special solutions is that of the creation of patient-specific lower jaw implants. They are designed based on CT data processed in a CAD system. Therefore auxiliary geometries have to be defined by the surgeon. Design and manufacture are thus performed on the implant producer's site. Our goal is to develop a software tool with which the doctor can define the auxiliary geometries after recording the CT data and can make these geometries directly available to the designing engineer.

2 Methods

The design of individualized lower jaw implants made of pure titanium is the subject of a current project financed by the Saxon Bank for Reconstruction and Development (SAB). The authors' partners in this interdisciplinary endeavor are doctors from the University Clinical Center Dresden and designing engineers from a product development firm. New technologies from medical image processing, Direct Manufacturing

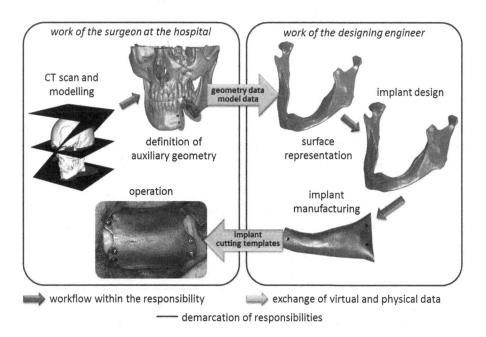

Fig. 1. Process chain for the manufacture of an individualized lower jaw implant

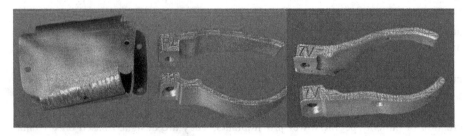

Fig. 2. Implant and cutting templates, manufactured with LaserCUSING®

(generative manufacturing) and Reverse Engineering are thus brought together. Below, we list the principal steps needed to create individualized implants (Fig. 1):

(1) Recording of the lower jaw region by means of computer tomography (CT) and generation of a surface model by means of the "marching cubes" algorithm

(2) Alignment of the lower jaw model in a defined co-ordinate system and definition of cutting planes (marking of the damaged area), fixing screws and dental implants

(3) Geometry reconstruction of removed part from the lower jaw; there are no limitations in any anatomical situation

(4) Surface representation of the lower jaw contour with follow-up design of implant and cutting templates (marking of the cutting position during operation)

(5) Preparation for generative production by means of LaserCUSING® [4] with subsequent manufacture of the implant and the cutting templates (Fig. 2)

(6) Preparation for generative production by means of LaserCUSING® with subsequent manufacture of the implant and the cutting templates.

3 Results

The product developed is the software tool "Kontito" (Fig. 3). Visualisation is based on XNA technology by Microsoft. This technology makes it possible to develop the tool quickly and simplifies its extension to applications that might be necessary in the future.

The functions are activated using a command manager, following a linear sequence of functions. Patient data are read in from the CT layered images (DICOM) or image data (TIFF, RAW etc.). Image artifacts of due to preexisting dental prostheses in the region of interest can corrupt the results of CT. After processing of the model data (such as cutting and clearing of triangles), the cutting planes are roughly aligned using three fixed surface points. Afterwards one can finely align the planes through shifting and rotation via mouse control. The accuracy depends from the resolution of the layered images during CT-procedure. In clinical situations the voxel size is between 1 and 2 mm. The error of design and manufacturing process is less than 0.01 mm.

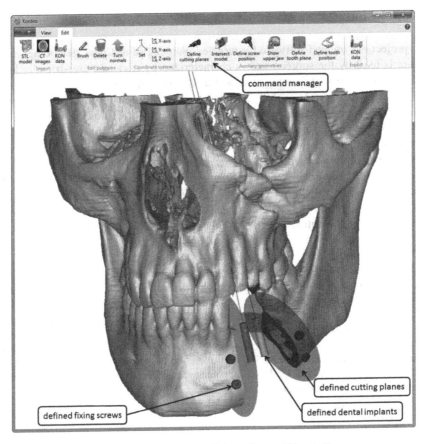

Fig. 3. User interface of the software "Kontito"

For the attachment of the mounting screws not only the intrinsic position is varied, but also the orientation, for instance in order to cover a greater region of the hard bone bed (corticalis) and thus to achieve better adhesion. Therefore it is possible to cut the model along the previously defined planes to make the inside area of the bone visible.

For broader functional integration into the lower jaw implant, position and orientation for dental implants that will be inserted are defined using the 3D model. To guarantee occlusion, orientation is taken from the arch contour of the lower jaw and the dental position of the upper jaw as well. Screws and tooth implants are shown in a simplified manner; the surgeon can freely select length and diameter. Thus, the surgeon can choose the preferred implant type from the wide variety of products on the market.

4   Conclusion

In the project, we created software for targeted planning of auxiliary geometries. The software is used by the surgeon and is characterized by easy and user-friendly handling. The software tool is integrated seamlessly into the entire process chain and makes possible an efficient exchange of design data between surgeon and designing engineer. The application has already been successfully tested using numerous 3D models of lower jaws taken from living minipigs, 20 cadavers of young pigs and on one human lower jaw. A validation of clinical effectiveness of this software-bridge will be a next step of our work.

In the future, additional auxiliary functions can be integrated. The plan is to simultaneously fade in both 3D model and CT layered images in the cutting region and to integrate algorithms to maintain occlusion between the lower- and upper jaws. Other options for the future are to use this application in the field of Augmented Reality (AR) or to embed other controls, such as a 3D mouse.

Acknowledgments. We acknowledge Dipl.-Ing. Gerd Engel, managing director of the product development company Hofmann & Engel Produktentwicklung GmbH in Boxdorf near Dresden, for his innovative ideas and his forward-looking decision to invest in an advanced laserCUS-ING® system at an early date. We also acknowledge Dipl.-Ing. Thomas Jahn, project manager in this scientific project in the company. Gerd Engel also contributed to the distribution of this modern technology in an industrial environment – and now for applications in the medical domain as well. We also acknowledge Dr. med. Jutta Markwardt from Department of Oral and Maxillofacial Surgery and Prof. Dr. Bernd Reitemeier from Department of Prosthetic Dentistry in Dresden for their innovative ideas.

References

1. Schöne, C., Stelzer, R., Sembdner, P., Markwardt, J., Reitemeier, B., Engel, G.: Individual contour adapted functional implant structures in titanium. In: Proceedings of the 21st CIRP Design Conference, KAIST, Korea, 27–29 March 2011. ISBN 978-89-89693-29-1
2. Schöne, C., Stelzer, R., Sembdner, P et al: Individual contour adapted functional implant structures in titanium. In: Proceedings of the 5th International Conference on Advanced Research and Rapid Prototyping (VRAP), Leiria, Portugal, 28 September–1 October 2011. ISBN: 978-0-415-68418-7
3. Bertol, L., Kindlein, W., Sembdner, P., Schöne, C., Stelzer, R.: Customized craniofacial implants: design and manufacture. In: Davim, P. (ed.) The Design and Manufacture of Medical Devices. Woodhead Publishing, Philadelphia (2012). ISBN 978-1-90756-872-5
4. Wohlers, T.: Rapid Prototyping and Manufacturing, State of the Industry. Wohlers Associates Inc, Colorado (2009). ISBN 0-9754429-5-3

Image-Based Bronchoscopy Navigation System Based on CT and C-arm Fluoroscopy

Teena Steger[✉], Klaus Drechsler, and Stefan Wesarg

Fraunhofer Institute for Computer Graphics Research, Fraunhoferstr. 5,
64283 Darmstadt, Germany
teena.steger@igd.fraunhofer.de
http://www.igd.fraunhofer.de

Abstract. Lung cancer diagnosis requires biopsy of airway tissue, which is mostly done by bronchoscopy. Although preoperative CT is available, intraoperatively only 2D information provided by the bronchoscopic camera and fluoroscopy is used. But, guidance of the bronchoscope to the target site would highly benefit from knowing the exact 3D position of the instrument inside the airways.

In this paper, we present a system for preoperative planning and intraoperative navigation during bronchoscopy. The preoperative components are automatic bronchial tree segmentation and skeletonization, semi-automatic tumor segmentation and a virtual fly-through simulation for planning purposes. During the intervention, we apply C-arm pose estimation using a marker plate on the patient table to align preoperative CT and intraoperative fluoroscopy. Thus, we can calculate the current 3D position of the bronchoscope inside the bronchial tree. Evaluation of the system components on patient CT and phantom fluoroscopy images showed promising results with high accuracy and robustness.

Keywords: Bronchoscopy · Intra-operative navigation · C-arm pose estimation · Segmentation · Fluoroscopy · CT

1 Introduction

Two steps are necessary to confidentially diagnose lung cancer: image-based examination of the lungs and biopsies of operatively extracted tissue samples. The second step is mostly done by bronchoscopy, i.e. guiding an endoscope through the airways to the targeted tumor site. Intraoperatively, only 2D images of the airways, endoscopic and fluoroscopic, are available. Obviously, providing a 3D view and the accurate position of the instrument inside the bronchial tree will enable faster and more accurate steering. Also, offering a preoperative virtual flight through the bronchial tree to the target lesion can significantly add value to the physician's preparation for the operation.

We present a navigational system for bronchoscopic interventions, which features preoperative simulation of the procedure for planning purposes and intraoperative guidance by giving the 3D position of the instrument inside the bronchial tree and, thus, providing orientation during bronchoscopy.

M. Erdt et al. (Eds.): CLIP 2013, LNCS 8361, pp. 15–22, 2014.
DOI: 10.1007/978-3-319-05666-1_3, © Springer International Publishing Switzerland 2014

2   Related Work

Endoscopy navigation systems mainly differ in their way to track the operational instruments during the intervention. For this, optical [1] or electromagnetic [2] sensors as well as purely image-based methods [3] are used. As optical tracking systems always come with a line-of-sight problem, they can only be employed with inflexible endoscopes, e.g. used during ENT-, CMF- and neuro surgery. Bronchoscopic navigation systems either rely on electromagnetic sensors fixed on the tip of a flexible bronchoscope [2] or apply image-based registration methods between the video frames acquired by the bronchoscopic camera and the preoperative CT [3]. Whereas the first solution behaves sensitively in the presence of ferromagnetic materials and needs to take respiratory motion and coughing into account, the second method is far from real-time capability and its accuracy is affected by bubbles in the airways, noise on the images and motion blur.

We propose using the C-arm images usually acquired during bronchoscopy and, thus, refrain from interfering with the physician's standard procedure. A similar approach is developed by *Xu et al.* in [4], where alignment between fluoroscopy and CT is found by image-based 2D/3D registration. But, this requires manual prepositioning after every C-arm movement, which can be quite time-consuming. Therefore, we rather apply C-arm pose estimation using only a specifically designed marker plate, which is placed on any C-arm patient table. Thus, our system can easily be integrated into common operation rooms. Although several marker-based C-arm pose estimation methods exist [5,6], none is suitable in shape, size and capture range for fluoroscopy images of the thoracic area acquired during bronchoscopy.

3   Materials and Methods

Our system consists of different parts, which we divide into preoperative and intraoperative components. Bronchial tree segmentation and skeletonization as well as tumor segmentation based on a CT are done preoperatively. The result of these steps enables a virtual "fly-through" through the airways to the target. Intraoperative components are a one-time patient-to-table image-based registration and C-arm pose estimation for each new fluoroscopy from a different pose. We use a specifically designed marker plate for this step. The two transformations, patient-to-table and table-to-C-arm, are used to estimate the current location of the bronchoscope inside the bronchial tree, provided the bronchoscope tip is visible on the fluoroscopy. Afterwards, this position can be visualized inside the correct bronchus and, thus, enhance the physician's view and orientation. Also, the previously segmented bronchial tree is virtually projected onto the fluoroscopy as a digitally reconstructed radiograph (DRR) to provide a more evident image of the airways. The following describes the individual components in detail.

3.1 Preoperative

Bronchial Tree Segmentation. Before the bronchoscopic intervention, a preoperative CT scan of the patient's lungs is acquired and examined. We provide a method for automatically extracting the airways from this CT scan in two steps: First, we find seed points inside the trachea. For this, we use a method described by Tschirren et al. [7]. The second step is a region growing-based segmentation using these seed points. Figure 1(a) shows an exemplary result of this segmentation and the utilized trachea seed points.

Skeletonization. The segmented bronchial tree needs to be reduced to a centerline representation. For this, we use our skeletonization method presented in [8]. Thus, the bronchi and bifurcations are transformed to centerlines (see Fig. 1(b)), which form the connected virtual guidance paths for the bronchoscope. These paths are important for the preoperative fly-through simulation as well as visualizing the intraoperative position of the bronchoscope inside the airways. For this, each voxel v of the skeleton is marked by a label l_v. Starting with labelling the bronchial tree root v_0 with $l_{v_0} = 1$, all neighbors v_1 are labelled with $l_{v_1} = l_{v_0} + 1$. This is recursively repeated for all skeleton voxels. A schematic result of this labelling is shown in Fig. 1(c).

Tumor Segmentation. A method published by Steger et al. [9] is applied for semi-automatic segmentation of lung lesions. Based on manually defining a single seed point inside the tumor, the surface is automatically segmented. This is done by a radial ray-based algorithm, which also takes local shape information into account. Figure 2(a) shows the radial rays starting from a seed point and the resulting segmentation surface. An exemplary lung lesion segmentation is shown in Fig. 2(b) in all three anatomical planes.

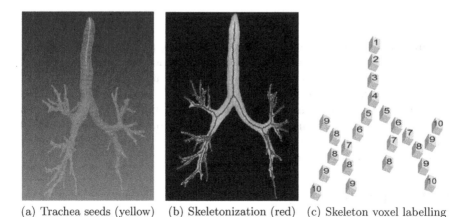

(a) Trachea seeds (yellow)   (b) Skeletonization (red)   (c) Skeleton voxel labelling

Fig. 1. Bronchial tree segmentation and skeletonization (Color figure online)

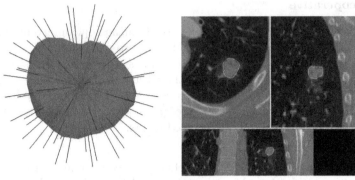

(a) Radial ray-based segmentation (b) Lung lesion segmentation result

Fig. 2. Tumor segmentation

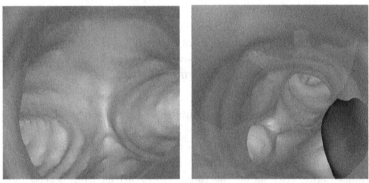

(a) Endoluminal view of bifurcation (b) Endoluminal view of target site

Fig. 3. Virtual fly-through with bronchoscopic guidance path (green) (Color figure online)

Virtual Fly-Through. Combining the results of the previous steps, bronchial tree and tumor segmentation as well as skeletonization, we now can produce a path from the trachea to the bronchus, which is adjacent to the targeted tumor. Afterwards, the physician can virtually "fly" alongside the generated path and view the bronchi and bifurcations on his way to the tumor. This can serve as a non-invasive examination as well as training or planning before the real intervention. Figure 3 shows exemplary views during a fly-through simulation at a bifurcation and at the targeted tumor site.

3.2   Intraoperative

Initial 2D/3D Registration. The transformation from patient to table needs to be calculated only once at the beginning of the procedure, as the patient

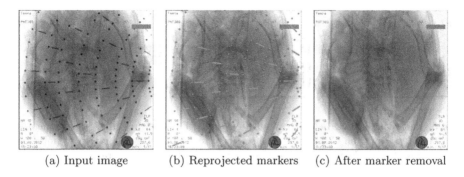

(a) Input image   (b) Reprojected markers   (c) After marker removal

Fig. 4. C-arm pose estimation and marker removal on X-ray of turkey cadaver

is sedated during the intervention and his or her position on the table rarely changes. This registration step is done semi-automatically, i.e. the user needs to provide a rough manual alignment, which serves as a starting point for the subsequent automatic intensity-based 2D/3D registration between intraoperative fluoroscopy and preoperative CT. We refrain from executing this step for every C-arm movement as it needs manual initialization and is by orders of magnitude slower in comparison to our marker-based C-arm pose estimation method, which is described in the next section.

C-arm Pose Estimation. Each time the physician acquires a new fluoroscopic image from a different position or angle, the transformation calculated at the beginning of the procedure changes. But, as the patient-to-table transformation stays almost steady, we only need to find the transformation between table and C-arm. For this purpose, we developed an acrylic marker plate, which can be easily fixed on any patient table (see Fig. 6(a)). The well-visible steel markers define a pattern, which allow unambiguous mapping between 3D source points on the plate and 2D image points on the fluoroscopy even after projection. For this, the projective invariant cross-ratio is deployed, which is defined on collinear points and concurrent lines. Details can be found in [10].

Marker Removal. Successful pose estimation enables reprojection of all visible markers onto the fluoroscopy (see Fig. 4(b)). Given their reprojected positions, these markers are removed using inpainting, which is exemplarily shown in Fig. 4(c). Thus, the markers do not disturb the physician's view. At the same time, the underlying anatomical structures are preserved for the most part.

Augmented Fluoroscopy. Knowing the non-varying transformation between patient and table and the varying transformation between table and C-arm, the relative position of the X-ray source and the patient's CT is computed. Using the beforehand segmented bronchial tree, a DRR of this binary volume can be generated. On this DRR, the airways are more evidently visible than on the real

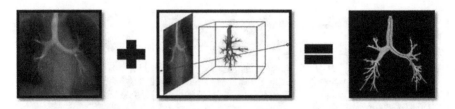

Fig. 5. Path calculation: *Left:* X-ray with overlayed DRR of bronchial tree segmentation. *Middle:* Ray from C-arm source through bronchial tree segmentation to point on fluoroscopy. *Right:* Calculated bronchoscope path inside bronchial tree.

fluoroscopy, which on the other hand clearly shows the bronchoscope. Overlaying virtual and real image provides additional information about the bronchoscope's position in relation to the airways. An exemplary DRR of a segmented bronchial tree can be seen in Fig. 5 (*left*).

Path Calculation. The bronchoscope tip is always well visible on the fluoroscopy and is selected manually. Then, a virtual ray from detector source to the selected pixel on the fluoroscopy image is defined. The intersecting bronchial tree segmentation voxels give the current 3D position of the bronchoscope tip. Given this position, we find the corresponding bronchus and the path to the trachea using the labelled skeleton of the bronchial tree (see Fig. 1(c)). This step is illustrated in Fig. 5.

4   Results

All preoperative and intraoperative components were integrated into one system for 3D bronchoscopy navigation, which we evaluated partly on clinical patient data and partly on phantom images. The following, describes these experiments and their results.

4.1   Preoperative

Bronchial tree segmentation was tested on the 30 chest CT scans provided by MICCAI EXACT'09 [11]. 25 bronchial trees were successfully segmented in 18.0 s on average and in 5 cases manual correction was be required due to leakage. A few segmentations were also skeletonized and used to generate artificial paths through the airways without a real tumor. Thus, we successfully tested our virtual fly-through. Tumor segmentation was tested on 10 chest CT scans provided by LIDC-IDRI [12][1] and the results visually inspected. All tumors were successfully segmented in 2.5 s on average.

---

[1] The authors acknowledge the National Cancer Institute and the Foundation for the National Institutes of Health and their critical role in the creation of the free publicly available LIDC/IDRI Database used in this study.

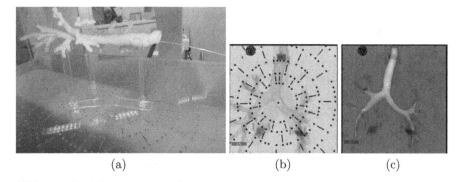

Fig. 6. Experimental set-up: *Left:* Airway model on marker plate in C-arm imaging field. *Middle:* Fluoroscopy of airway model and marker plate. *Right:* Fluoroscopy with removed markers and accurately overlayed DRR of bronchial tree segmentation

4.2   Intraoperative

The intraoperative components were tested with a hollow bronchial tree model segmented from a thorax CT volume using our method and made of transparent polyurethane. First, we acquired a high-resolution CT scan of this model. Then, we placed the bronchial tree on the marker plate, which on its part was placed on a patient table (see Fig. 6(a)). Using a Ziehm flat-detector C-arm, 41 X-ray images from typical positions and angles were acquired (see Fig. 6(b)). After initial patient-to-table alignment on the first image, C-arm pose estimation was executed on the following images, of which 20 were acquired by translations in x- ([−20 cm; 20 cm]), y- ([−15 cm; 15 cm]) and z-direction ([67 cm; 52 cm]) and 20 by rotations around the transversal ([−15°; 15°]) and longitudinal ([−20°; 20°]) axis. Afterwards, all visible markers were removed from the images by inpainting (see Fig. 6(c)). DRRs using the estimated poses and the initial patient-to-table transformation were generated and overlayed on the fluoroscopic images (see Fig. 6(c)). Thus, we were able to visually inspect the quality of the results. All translated images were correctly reprojected. Only two rotated images resulted in inaccurate pose estimations. As the overlap between reprojected and original branches were insufficient, they did not pass visual inspection. On the whole, our method proved fully satisfying accuracy and robustness for translations and rotations. On average pose estimation took 1.1 s on each image. Path calculation using a manually selected point on an imaged bronchus was accomplished in all cases with successful and accurate pose estimation.

5   Conclusions

A navigation system for preoperative simulation and intraoperative instrument guidance during bronchoscopy was presented and evaluated. We use C-arm pose estimation on a marker plate for aligning CT to fluoroscopy and, thus, determining the instrument's location inside the airways. Hence, the system does not need any optical or electromagnetic tracking devices, which makes it easy to integrate in typical operation rooms without interfering with the common clinical procedure. It was thoroughly tested on thorax CT scans and real C-arm images of a bronchial tree model and delivered promising results. The next step will be clinical trial of the whole system.

References

1. Hong, J., et al.: Endoscopic image overlay surgical navigation using augmented and virtual reality technologies. In: ASCC, pp. 574–578 (2011)
2. Reichl, T., et al.: Real-time motion compensation for EM bronchoscope tracking with smooth output – ex-vivo validation. In: SPIE Medical Imaging (2012)
3. Deguchi, D., et al.: Selective image similarity measure for bronchoscope tracking based on image registration. MIA **13**, 621–633 (2009)
4. Xu, D., et al.: Single-view 2D/3D registation for X-ray guided bronchoscopy. In: IEEE ISBI, ISBI'10, pp. 233–236. IEEE Press (2010)
5. Kainz, B., et al.: Fast marker based C-arm pose estimation. MICCAI **11**, 652–659 (2008)
6. Fallavollita, P., Burdette, C., Song, D.Y., Abolmaesumi, P., Fichtinger, G.: C-arm tracking by intensity-based registration of a fiducial in prostate brachytherapy. In: Navab, N., Jannin, P. (eds.) IPCAI 2010. LNCS, vol. 6135, pp. 45–55. Springer, Heidelberg (2010)
7. Tschirren, J., et al.: Airway segmentation framework for clinical environments. In: Brown, M., et al. (eds.) MICCAI Workshop on Pulmonary Image Analysis, London, UK, pp. 227–238 (2009)
8. Drechsler, K., et al.: Dimension reduction based on centroids for multimodal anatomical landmark-based 3D/2D registration of coronary angiograms. In: IVAPP (2010)
9. Steger, S., Sakas, G.: FIST: fast interactive segmentation of tumors. In: Yoshida, H., Sakas, G., Linguraru, M.G. (eds.) Abdominal Imaging, MICCAI'11. LNCS, vol. 7029, pp. 125–132. Springer, Heidelberg (2012)
10. Steger, T., et al.: Marker detection evaluation by phantom and cadaver experiments for C-arm pose estimation pattern. In: SPIE Medical Imaging, pp. 86711V–86711V-9 (2013)
11. Lo, P., et al.: Extraction of airways from CT (EXACT'09). IEEE Trans. Med. Imaging **31**(11), 2093–2107 (2012)
12. Armato 3rd, S., et al.: The lung image database consortium (LIDC): ensuring the integrity of expert-defined "truth". Acad. Radiol. **14**(12), 1455–1463 (2007)

Path Planning for Multi-port Lateral Skull Base Surgery Based on First Clinical Experiences

Meike Becker[1]([⊠]), Stefan Hansen[2], Stefan Wesarg[3], and Georgios Sakas[1]

[1] Interactive Graphics Systems Group, TU Darmstadt, Darmstadt, Germany
meike.becker@gris.tu-darmstadt.de
[2] Department of Oto-Rhino-Laryngology, Düsseldorf University Hospital,
Düsseldorf, Germany
[3] Cognitive Computing and Medical Imaging, Fraunhofer IGD, Darmstadt, Germany

Abstract. Our research project investigates a multi-port minimally-traumatic approach for lateral skull base surgery, where the surgical target shall be reached through up to three drill canals. For this purpose, an accurate path planning is crucial. In the present work, we propose a semi-automatic path planning approach for multi-port minimally-traumatic lateral skull base surgery. The best path combinations are automatically determined by optimizing the angles and distance buffers of the drill canals. We compare the automatically computed path combinations for 20 data sets to those selected manually by two different clinicians. The experiments prove that we can adequately reproduce the clinicians' choice.

Keywords: Path planning · Minimally-traumatic surgery · Multi-port

1 Introduction

Lateral skull base surgery is one of the more complex surgeries due to the small size and narrow location of the anatomical structures. Possible interventions are a cochlear implant, drug-delivery or tumor dissection. The main challenge is not to damage any critical structures such as blood vessels, the cochlea or the facial nerve. So far the common clinical practice is largely traumatic (see Fig. 1(a)). The surgeon mills away a huge part of the bone and exposes all critical structures in order to ensure their intactness.

Our research project investigates a multi-port approach for minimally-traumatic lateral skull base surgery. The objective of the multi-port technique is to use up to three drill canals leading from the skull surface to the surgical site: one for the instrument, one for the endoscope and one for material removal or for a second instrument. In this case the surgeon will not be able to rely on the exposed structures for orientation anymore. Hence, an accurate patient-specific planning based on image data is crucial.

In the following, we present a semi-automatic path planning approach for multi-port minimally-traumatic lateral skull base surgery. For optimization we

M. Erdt et al. (Eds.): CLIP 2013, LNCS 8361, pp. 23–30, 2014.
DOI: 10.1007/978-3-319-05666-1_4, © Springer International Publishing Switzerland 2014

use an objective function that combines two features: the angles between the three paths and the remaining distance buffer of each of the three drill canals (see Fig. 2). Only the target and the center and size of the set of possible entry points have to be determined by the clinician. In the experiments section, we automatically compute path combinations for 20 computed tomography (CT) data sets and compare them to the manual choice of two clinicians.

2   Related Work

There is ongoing research on drilling a single path to a surgical target in the temporal bone: Several cadaveric studies have shown the feasibility of a single drill path to the cochlea and the petrous apex [3,11] and Labadie et al. [7] have conducted a clinical validation study for single-port cochlear implant surgery. Our research project now investigates a multi-port approach. To the best of our knowledge, no such technique has yet been described in scientific publications.

Since the structures in the temporal bone are very small, high accuracy is needed. Therefore, an accurate planning is crucial. Most of the path planning methods define a set of constraints and classify them into two categories: hard constraints, which have to be satisfied (e.g. the intactness of critical structures) and soft constraints, which are optimized (e.g. the distance to critical structures). In other areas, such as abdominal and neurosurgery, several approaches for planning a single path do exist. Essert et al. [5] for example presented a geometric constraint solver for computing the optimal placement of an electrode for deep brain stimulation. Seitel et al. [10] compute possible insertion zones for needle placement in radio frequency ablation and use the concept of pareto-optimality to allow for a weight-independent rating of the trajectories.

In contrast, research in the context of lateral skull base surgery is rare and focuses on a single port. Al-Marzouqi et al. [1] present an atlas-based approach where they transfer a manually placed trajectory from an atlas to the CT data of the current patient using registration. Noble et al. [8] state that this trajectory is not guaranteed to be safe (i.e. to avoid critical structures) and effective (i.e. to reach the round window at a certain angle and position). Therefore, they propose a monte-carlo-simulation based approach to optimize such a given trajectory with respect to safety and effectiveness while accounting for the drill positioning error.

Eilers et al. [4] also base their approach on the concept of hard and soft constraints. First of all, they eliminate all trajectories which would damage a critical structure or would not reach the cochlea at a certain angle. Then they optimize the weighted distance to the critical structures. Riechmann et al. [9] propose to use a drill canal with a user-defined radius which is freely manoeuvrable. The movement is blocked if a collision with a critical structure occurs. Their approach allows to place several of these canals individually but does not automatically optimize any features.

All of the previous methods are designed for using a single port, with the sole exception of Riechmann et al. whose method permits manually placing

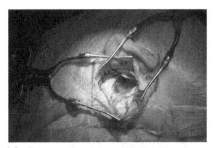

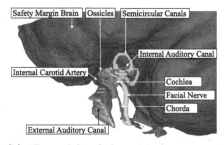

(a) Conventional surgery leading to a high traumatization of the patient.

(b) 3D models of the critical structures loaded into the planning tool.

Fig. 1. In addition to conventional surgery (a), where planning takes place in the surgeon's mind, we propose a multi-port approach, where planning is computer-aided (b).

several individual canals, but without automatically optimizing any features. The present work, in contrast, is focused on an automated multi-port approach.

3 Methods

The planning tool we are currently developing is based on the Simulation Open Framework Architecture [6] and has been partly described in [2].

Preprocessing. Since the planning is patient specific, we first of all have to extract the critical structures from the image data of the patient. The following structures have been declared critical by the clinicians and are visualized in Fig. 1(b): facial nerve, chorda, semicircular canals, cochlea, ossicles, internal carotid artery, internal auditory canal, external auditory canal and a safety margin for the dura, which is the outermost of the three layers surrounding the brain. The critical structures are currently labeled manually in the CT data. Then the 3D models are extracted and loaded into the planning tool as a 3D scene.

Planning. First, the clinician defines a target point t in the CT data. Then, he or she roughly selects a set of obvious candidate entry points in the 3D scene by clicking on the surface of the 3D model of the cranial bone. All triangle center points of the cranial bone's mesh within a certain distance to this center point are chosen as candidate entry points. There is a straight path p from each candidate entry point $s \in \mathbb{R}^3$ to the target point t (see Fig. 2 for illustration). For each combination of three paths p_1, p_2 and p_3, we have three angles: the angle $\alpha_{12} = \angle(p_1, p_2)$ between path p_1 and p_2, $\alpha_{23} = \angle(p_2, p_3)$ and $\alpha_{31} = \angle(p_3, p_1)$ respectively. Further, for each drill canal defined by path p and radius r, the distance buffer b denotes the remaining minimum distance to the critical structures.

Our goal is now to determine out of the set of all candidate paths, a combination c of three paths, where the three angles between the paths and the remaining

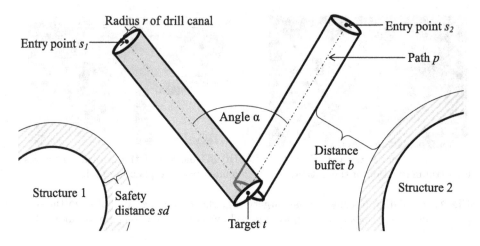

Fig. 2. Illustration of the path planning parameters for two drill canals.

distance buffer b of each drill canal are as large as possible. The two features have been chosen in agreement with the clinicians. The angles are maximized in order to minimize the intersection of the drill canals.

For the planning step, we have *technical* parameters and *medical* parameters. The technical process-related parameters include the minimal radius r of the drill canal, the uncertainty of the drill and the safety distance sd to the critical structures which has to be absolutely maintained due to uncertainty of image acquisition and segmentation (see Fig. 2 for illustration). The medical parameters consist of a global minimum threshold α_{thresh} for the angle between the paths and a threshold b_{thresh} for the distance buffer to the critical structures.

As in the related work, our approach consists of two steps. First, we eliminate all paths which would damage a critical structure in regard to the technical parameters. This is done using exhaustive search. The resulting feasible paths are then color coded according to the size of the remaining distance buffer b (see Fig. 3(a)).

Second, we calculate the best combination of three paths out of the set of feasible paths. This is done by optimizing the angles and the distance buffers between the three paths as follows: We first normalize the feature values and then maximize the objective function

$$f(c) = (1 - w_b) \cdot (\alpha_{12} + \alpha_{23} + \alpha_{31}) + w_b \cdot (b_1 + b_2 + b_3) \qquad (1)$$

over all possible combinations c, where $w_b \geq 0$ describes the weight for the distance buffer and $\alpha_{12}, \alpha_{23}, \alpha_{31} \geq \alpha_{\text{thresh}}$ and $b_1, b_2, b_3 \geq b_{\text{thresh}}$ have to be satisfied. The way of choosing the parameters w_b, α_{thresh} and b_{thresh} will be explained in Sect. 4. For optimization, we use exhaustive search. Due to the discretization of the search space the exhaustive search is sufficient.

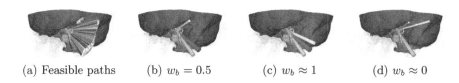

(a) Feasible paths   (b) $w_b = 0.5$ (c) $w_b \approx 1$ (d) $w_b \approx 0$

Fig. 3. Out of a set of feasible paths (a), a combination of three paths is computed. Examples of different weights are shown in (b) - (d) for the target IAC.

4   Evaluation

Settings. All of our experiments are retrospective and are based on the same data of 20 CT data sets acquired with a standard CT scanner and an average resolution of $0.19 \times 0.19 \times 0.39 \, \text{mm}^3$. Three different target structures have been considered: the round window (RW), the internal auditory canal (IAC) and the petrous apex (PA). Since reasonable values for the parameters are still being researched, the following technical parameters have been fixed in accordance with the clinicians and without loss of generality: the minimal drill radius r has been set to 0.5 mm, the drill uncertainty and safety distance sd have been set to 0. The medical parameters α_{thresh} and b_{thresh} are determined empirically as described below.

Experiments. Since the multi-port technique is not yet in clinical use, we do not know what the best combination of paths for a multi-port approach is. Therefore, in a previous work [2], a clinician used the planning tool to manually select a combination of three paths out of a set of feasible paths. Herefrom, we have derived first conditions for defining a good combination of paths.

The experiments for the present work were conducted in three steps. First of all, a second clinician repeated the manual choice of a good combination of paths based on the same data sets and parameters in order to account for inter-observer variability. Based on those two manual choices of path combinations, we dimensioned our system and empirically determined the medical parameters α_{thresh} and b_{thresh} for the automatic computation. As reported in [2], the feature values are different for every of the three target structures. For example, the angles to be applied for surgery of the PA are smaller than those for surgery of the IAC and the RW. Hence, we assume three different medical parameter settings which are specific for each of the three target structures.

In a second step, we automatically computed path combinations for the same 20 data sets, using the optimization method as described in Sect. 3. Here, we considered three different cases: uniform weights ($w_b = 0.5$), weighing only the distance buffer ($w_b \approx 1$) and weighing only the angle ($w_b \approx 0$). We do not use equality for $w_b \approx 1$ and $w_b \approx 0$ in order to be able to differentiate for example between two combinations having the same angle but different distance buffers, if the case is $w_b \approx 0$. One example on how the different weights influence the result is given in Fig. 3.

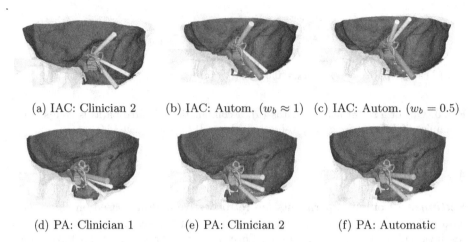

(a) IAC: Clinician 2   (b) IAC: Autom. ($w_b \approx 1$)   (c) IAC: Autom. ($w_b = 0.5$)

(d) PA: Clinician 1   (e) PA: Clinician 2   (f) PA: Automatic

Fig. 4. Examples of path combinations. In the first row, we see that the automatically computed combination with $w_b \approx 1$ (b) is similar to the choice of the clinician (a), while using $w_b = 0.5$ (c) represents a feasible alternative. In the second row, we observe that variability also exists between the clinicians' choices.

In a third step, we presented the five combinations (clinician 1, clinician 2, $w_b \approx 0$, $w_b = 0.5$ and $w_b \approx 1$) for all 20 data sets blindly and randomized to a third clinician for validation, and the clinician rated them all.

Results. Good rates were achieved for the target structure RW, where at least one automatically computed combination was comparable to the clinicians' choice. For the targets IAC and PA, it turned out that the empirically computed value α_{thresh} was too low. Hence, we refined the thresholds by excluding the manually chosen path combinations rated lowest by clinician 3 and recomputed the medical parameters from the remaining data sets. Then, we repeated the automatic calculation of the path combinations for the targets IAC and PA.

We visually assessed the results of the automatic computation for all 20 data sets and found that in all 20 cases at least one automatically computed combination was comparable to the clinicians' manual choices, a fact which has been confirmed by the third clinician. Examples are shown in Fig. 4. For the given parameter settings, in some cases the uniform weights performed better and in other cases weighing the distance buffer led to better results. In most cases, weighing the angle led to unsatisfying results. At least one of the three automatically computed path combinations show characteristics described in [2]: For the target IAC, one drill canal goes through the upper semicircular canal. In most cases, the other two canals pass on the posterior side of the facial nerve, while in the remaining cases, one passes posterior and one anterior to the facial nerve. For the RW, all canals pass between the facial nerve and the external auditory canal. Again, for the target PA it is difficult to find any common characteristics among the available data sets.

Table 1. Quantitative results for each target structure for the minimum angle $\alpha_{min} = \min(\alpha_{12}, \alpha_{23}, \alpha_{31})$ and minimum distance buffer $b_{min} = \min(b_1, b_2, b_3)$ of the drill path combinations. Mean, standard deviation (SD) and minimum over the 20 data sets are shown.

α_{min} (in $^\circ$)	IAC Mean		Min	RW Mean		Min	PA Mean		Min
Clinician 1	16	(SD: 6)	9	23	(SD: 9)	8	10	(SD: 5)	4
Clinician 2	14	(SD: 7)	9	21	(SD: 8)	11	10	(SD: 4)	4
Automatic	18	(SD: 7)	10	18	(SD: 16)	9	12	(SD: 5)	6

b_{min} (in mm)	Mean		Min	Mean		Min	Mean		Min
Clinician 1	0.7	(SD: 0.3)	0.3	0.7	(SD: 0.2)	0.3	0.7	(SD: 0.4)	0.2
Clinician 2	0.8	(SD: 0.2)	0.3	0.9	(SD: 0.3)	0.4	0.8	(SD: 0.4)	0.3
Automatic	0.7	(SD: 0.3)	0.3	1.0	(SD: 0.4)	0.4	0.5	(SD: 0.4)	0.3

As shown in Table 1, the quantitative results for the minimum angle and distance buffer of the path combinations are also comparable within the standard deviation.

Discussion. The experiments show that the automatic computation of path combinations achieves results comparable to the manual choice of the clinicians. During the experiments, we identified an additional constraint: In CT data, the facial nerve is indirectly visible due to its bony canal within the temporal bone. However, the extratemporal part is not visible and hence has not been segmented for the experiments. As a consequence, the planning tool does not guarantee the intactness of the extratemporal part of the facial nerve. For each target structure, there were one to two patients for whom the extratemporal part of the facial nerve would either be damaged or was not sure to be avoided. Therefore, the intactness of the extratemporal part of the facial nerve has to be included as an additional constraint in the future. This may be done by explicitly eliminating all paths in the risk area between the facial nerve and the external auditory canal and below the end of the segmentation of the facial nerve. Another possibility would be to find means to segment the extratemporal part of the facial nerve in the image data.

Furthermore, we detected a high inter-observer variability in the choice of the path combinations. Therefore, showing different possibilities, for example using different weights as we did, is recommendable in order to allow the clinician to make a choice according to his or her individual preference.

5   Conclusion

In the present work, we introduce an approach for semi-automatic path planning for multi-port lateral skull base surgery. A combination of up to three drill canals is determined by optimizing an objective function based on the angles between the paths and the remaining distance buffer of the drill canals. In our experiments, we automatically computed path combinations for 20 data sets and compared them to the manual choices of two clinicians. The experiments show that we can adequately reproduce the clinicians' choice. During the experiments, we identified a new constraint concerning the protection of the extratemporal part of the facial nerve which will have to be incorporated in the future. With our planning tool, we aim at supporting the surgeon concerned with research on multi-port lateral skull base surgery with the goal of a prospective use.

Acknowledgments. This work has been funded by the *German Research Foundation (DFG)*: FOR 1585; FE 431/13-1.

References

1. Al-Marzouqi, H., Noble, J.H., Warren, F.M., Labadie, R.F., Fitzpatrick, J.M., Dawant, B.: Planning a safe drilling path for cochlear implantation surgery using image registration techniques. In: Proceedings of the SPIE 6509, Medical Imaging 2007: Visualization and Image-Guided Procedures, pp. 331–339 (2007)
2. Becker, M., Gutbell, R., Stenin, I., Wesarg, S.: Towards automatic path planning for multi-port minimally-traumatic lateral skull base surgery. In: Drechsler, K., Erdt, M., Linguraru, M.G., Oyarzun Laura, C., Sharma, K., Shekhar, R., Wesarg, S. (eds.) CLIP 2012. LNCS, vol. 7761, pp. 59–66. Springer, Heidelberg (2013)
3. Bell, B., Stieger, C., Gerber, N., Arnold, A., Nauer, C., Hamacher, V., Kompis, M., Nolte, L., Caversaccio, M., Weber, S.: A self-developed and constructed robot for minimally invasive cochlear implantation. Acta Otolaryngol. **132**, 355–360 (2012)
4. Eilers, H., Baron, S., Ortmaier, T., Heimann, B., Baier, C., Rau, T.S., Leinung, M., Majdani, O.: Navigated, robot assisted drilling of a minimally invasive cochlear access. In: International Conference on Mechatronics. pp. 259–266. Springer (2009) NULL
5. Essert, C., Haegelen, C., Lalys, F., Abadie, A., Jannin, P.: Automatic computation of electrode trajectories for deep brain stimulation: a hybrid symbolic and numerical approach. Int. J. Comput. Assist. Radiol. Surg. **7**(4), 517–532 (2012)
6. Faure, F., Duriez, C., Delingette, H., et al.: Sofa: a multi-model framework for interactive physical simulation. In: Payan, Y. (ed.) Soft Tissue Biomechanical Modeling for Computer Assisted Surgery. Studies in Mechanobiology, Tissue Engineering and Biomaterials, vol. 11, pp. 283–321. Springer, Heidelberg (2012)
7. Labadie, R.F., Balachandran, R., Mitchell, J., Noble, J.H., Majdani, O., Haynes, D., Bennett, M., Dawant, B.M., Fitzpatrick, J.M.: Clinical validation study of percutaneous cochlear access using patient customized micro-stereotactic frames. Otol. Neurotol. **31**(1), 94–99 (2010)
8. Noble, J.H., Majdani, O., Labadie, R.F., Dawant, B., Fitzpatrick, J.M.: Automatic determination of optimal linear drilling trajectories for cochlear access accounting for drill-positioning error. Int. J. Med. Rob. Comput. Assist. Surg. **6**(3), 281–290 (2010)
9. Riechmann, M., Lohnstein, P.U., Raczkowsky, J., Klenzner, T., Schipper, J., Wörn, H.: Identifying access paths for endoscopic interventions at the lateral skull base. Int. J. Comput. Assist. Radiol. Surg. **3**, 249–250 (2008)
10. Seitel, A., Engel, M., Sommer, C., et al.: Computer-assisted trajectory planning for percutaneous needle insertions. Med. Phys. **38**(6), 3246–3260 (2011)
11. Wanna, G., Balachandran, R., Majdani, O., Mitchell, J., Labadie, R.: Percutaneous access to the petrous apex in vitro using customized micro-stereotactic frames based on image-guided surgical technology. Acta Otolaryngol. **130**, 458–463 (2010)

On-Line Lumen Centre Detection in Gastrointestinal and Respiratory Endoscopy

Carles Sánchez[(✉)], Jorge Bernal, Debora Gil, and F. Javier Sánchez

Computer Vision Centre and Computer Science Department,
Campus Universitat Autònoma de Barcelona, 08193 Bellaterra, Barcelona, Spain
{csanchez,jbernal,debora,javier}@cvc.uab.cat

Abstract. We present in this paper a novel lumen centre detection for gastrointestinal and respiratory endoscopic images. The proposed method is based on the appearance and geometry of the lumen, which we defined as the darkest image region which centre is a hub of image gradients. Experimental results validated on the first public annotated gastro-respiratory database prove the reliability of the method for a wide range of images (with precision over 95 %).

Keywords: Lumen centre detection · Bronchoscopy · Colonoscopy

1 Introduction

Optical endoscopy is used nowadays to examine the interior of hollow organs or cavities of the body. These methods consist of introducing an instrument called endoscope which has a light source and a camera mounted on it to observe the particular organ. There is a recent trend on developing intelligent systems for endoscopy which aim at providing additional information to the procedure by analysing image content. The most immediate applications of these systems are: the on-line assistance in the diagnosis, to provide a complete endoluminal scene description (intervention time) or quality assessment (post-intervention).

The objective of this work is the characterization of the lumen centre in bronchoscopy and colonoscopy videos. Lumen centre detection can be useful for several applications such as: (1) scene description; (2) calculation of the navigation path or (3) seed of lumen segmentation algorithms.

A main challenge is to cope with the large variability in lumen appearance across images types and acquisitions. Such variability is related to differences in acquisition and illumination conditions and make it difficult to define a model of appearance common to colon and bronchi. Figure 1 shows different lumen appearances in bronchi (Fig. 1(a,b)) and colon (Fig. 1(c,d)) procedures. The lumen in bronchoscopy is enclosed by the concentric tracheobronchial rings and it is usually centred in the image. This is not the case of colon lumen which might be in any part of the image related on the navigation differences.

The majority of the relevant work in lumen localization and detection is related to gastrointestinal image analysis. Under the assumptions that the largest

M. Erdt et al. (Eds.): CLIP 2013, LNCS 8361, pp. 31–38, 2014.
DOI: 10.1007/978-3-319-05666-1_5, © Springer International Publishing Switzerland 2014

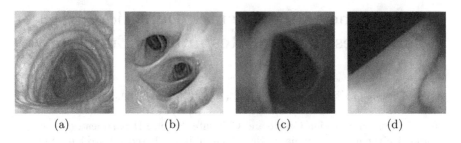

     (a)   (b)   (c)   (d)

Fig. 1. Examples of variability in lumen appearance: single (a) and multiple (b) bronchoscopy image; centred (c) and biased (d) colonoscopy image.

dark blob of the images usually correspond to lumen [1] and it is always present in the images [2], there are several works that segment the lumen using a region growing approach over the image grey level [3]. These approaches are accurate as far as the initial seed for the region growing is placed inside the luminal area and their performance decrease in the presence of shadows or low contrast images. Recent approaches use contrast changes to account for local differences in image intensity. For instance, the authors in [4] characterize the luminal region in wireless capsule videos by means of Haar features followed by a supervised boosting for detecting the probability of having the lumen in a given frame. A main drawback for its application to standard bronchospcopy procedures is that its usual central navigation illuminates the luminal area and, thus, reduces contrast changes (compare images in Fig. 1(a) and (b)).

A common limitation is that most methods can not handle having more than one lumen in an image, which is quite frequent in bronchoscopy videos. The recent approach in [5] detects multiple lumen areas by using mean shift. Although it provides information about multiple lumen, it might fail in the absence of any luminal area and it has a high computational cost not suitable for its use in intervention time. Other approaches for multiple lumen detection in bronchoscopy [6,7] are semi-automatic procedures which are applied off-line. Finally, up to our knowledge, there is no public annotated database of lumen regions (for, both, bronchoscopy and colonoscopy videos) allowing the comparison of the performance of different methods. This constitutes a major flaw for the development of generic algorithms able to achieve accurate results in a wide range of images.

This paper addresses two main points in the context of lumen characterization in endoscopy videos. First, we present a lumen centre detection method that can be used for a wide range of endoscopic images, covering single and multiple lumens. The proposed method is inspired on the work in tracheal ring segmentation presented in [8] and combines appearance and geometric features of the lumen that are present in both bronchoscopy and colonoscopy frames. Second, we present a manually annotated database, which includes representative cases of colonoscopy and bronchoscopy videos, along with a validation protocol. The rest of the paper is structured as follows: our lumen centre detection method is

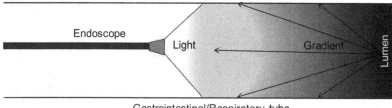

Fig. 2. Model of appearance of the lumen based on the illumination.

presented in Sect. 2. We introduce our validation protocol including the description of the annotated database in Sect. 3. Results are reported in Sect. 4 and conclusions in Sect. 5.

2   Lumen Centre Detection

Our processing scheme consists of three different stages: (1) Image preprocessing; (2) Calculation of Lumen Energy Maps (LEMs) and (3) Obtention of the centre points. Specific details about the preprocessing steps can be found in [9]. The central point of our method, the calculation of LEM maps, is based on a model of appearance of the lumen and it has been designed to overcome the limitations of existing approaches. Finally the obtention of the centre point uses unsupervisded learning over a training set to provide the likelihood of a pixel to be inside the lumen. The local maxima of such likelihood map are our lumen centres.

2.1   Model of Appearance of the Lumen

In order to build our model of appearance of the lumen we will lean on a graphical scheme of how endoscopy images are generated, shown in Fig. 2. As illustrated in Fig. 2, the amount of light that falls on the scene decreases approximately according to the square of the distance between the light source and each 3D point. Consequently the farthest parts of the image, such as the lumen, are poorly lighted. The fact that the amount of light increases from the centre of the lumen outwards allows to incorporate geometric gradient-based features to our characterization of the lumen. Our model of appearance for lumen uses the former cues to characterize the lumen centre as the dark region of the image which centre is the hub of image gradients. These two cues are used to develop our two LEM maps algorithms which are described next.

2.2   LEM Maps

We present here two different Lumen Energy Maps. The first one, **Directed Gradient Accumulation (DGA)**, is based on the idea that the lumen centre is the source of all image gradients whereas the second, **Dark Region Identification (DRI)**, exploits the fact that lumen region tends to be the darker part of the image.

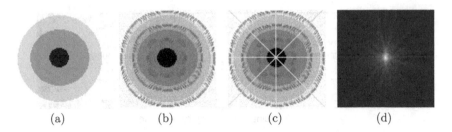

(a)   (b)   (c)   (d)

Fig. 3. Graphical explanation of DGA algorithm: Original synthetic image (a); Corresponding gradient vectors superimposed to the image (b); Example of the extension of gradient vector lines (c), and resulting DGA accumulation map (d).

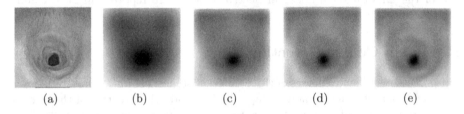

(a)   (b)   (c)   (d)   (e)

Fig. 4. Graphical explanation of DRI algorithm: Original bronchoscopy image (a); Smoothed images with σ: 1/8 (b); 1/16 (c); 1/24 (d); 1/32 (e).

DGA value for each point is calculated as the number of gradient-directed lines that cross it. These lines have the same direction than the gradient and they are created by extending gradient lines to cover the whole frame. If a given image point is at the centre of a tubular structure, by Phong's illumination model, image normal lines will accumulate around this point. It follows that DGA achieves maximum values at either darker (i.e. lumen) or brighter (i.e. specular highlights, polyps) regions. The synthetic images in Fig. 3 illustrate how DGA works. In this example all gradient vectors are directed from the centre of the image (darkest part) to the brightest external part and, thus, DGA maximum response corresponds to the centre of the image (Fig. 3(d)).

DRI maps are calculated by applying a smoothing using a gaussian kernel which σ is related to the scale of the lumen and it is determined using a training set. The response to DRI enhances dark values and, thus, the lumen region. Figure 4 shows the output of DRI for several scales. Note that as we decrease the scale we go from having a big dark blob (Fig. 4(b)) to a smaller one which matches better the lumen region (Fig. 4(e)).

2.3 Centre Point Characterization

The 2D feature space given by (DGA,DRI) characterizes several elements of the endoluminal scene. In particular, pixels belonging to the lumen have a low value of DRI and a high DGA value, polyps have high DGA and DRI and structures like folds and rings (which generate shadows) have low DGA and DRI values. The

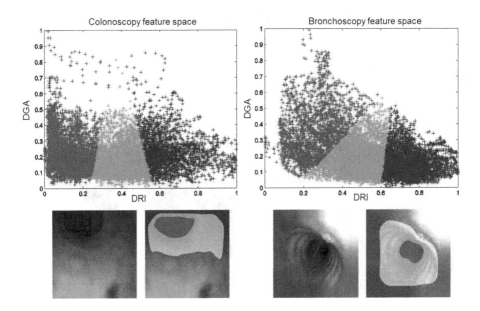

Fig. 5. Adequation of our feature space to bronchoscopy and colonoscopy examples.

partition of the feature space into this three classes is obtained by unsupervised k-means clustering over a training set. In order to have comparable values, the output of both LEM maps has been normalized in $[0, 1]$ range. This normalization has been obtained by means of the maximum and minimum values achieved for the training set.

The distance of a pixel to the borders given by the clustering defines a likelihood map of its belonging to the each of the classes. In our application this border has been approximated by a linear plane of origin (DRI_0, DGA_0) and normal direction (V_{DRI}, V_{DGA}), so, for each feature point (DRI, DGA) its likelihood map LK is defined by:

$$LK(DRI, DGA) = (DRI - DRI_0)V_{DRI} + (DGA - DGA_0)V_{DGA} \quad (1)$$

A threshold, Th_{LK}, on LK determines those points having a larger likelihood of belonging to a given class. We obtain the optimal Th_{LK} value as the maximum value of the ROC curve [10] corresponding to lumen segmentation for the training set. This stage has been applied separately for bronchoscopy and colonoscopy images. Figure 5 shows our feature spaces obtained for each type of images.

Finally to calculate to the lumen centre we proceed as follows: for the case of colonoscopy videos, as there is only one lumen per image, we take the best candidate inside the lumen region cluster. On the other hand for bronchoscopy we take all the local maxima that we may find inside the lumen cluster.

Table 1. Description of lumen database.

Index	Type	Resolution
1–100	Bronchoscopy[a]	$[144 \times 144, 288 \times 288, 186 \times 186]$
101–200	Colonoscopy[b]	$[500 \times 577]$
201–225	Bronchoscopy(15 multi-lumen and 10 no lumen)[a]	$[144 \times 144, 288 \times 288, 186 \times 186]$
226–250	Colonoscopy (no-lumen)[b]	$[144 \times 144, 288 \times 288, 186 \times 186]$

[a]Bellvitge Hospital Barcelona
[b]Beaumont and St. Vincents Hospistal Dublin

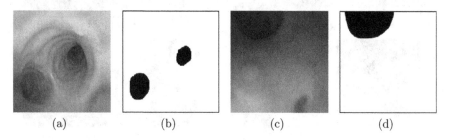

(a)   (b)   (c)   (d)

Fig. 6. Examples of images from our database: bronchoscopy image (a) and its ground truth (b); colonoscopy image (c) and its ground truth (d).

3   The Annotated Database and Validation Protocol

In order to be useful for validating a wide range of algorithms, an annotated database should fulfill the following requirements: (1) It should contain examples of frames with lumen from both bronchoscopy and colonoscopy videos; (2) The selected frames should be different enough in order to have the maximum variability available of lumen appearance; (3) The database should also contain examples of frames both with multiple lumen (bronchoscopy) and without lumen. Taking these constraints into account we have built up a database of 250 images[1] extracted from 15 and 20 sequences of colonoscopy and bronchoscopy respectively. Table 1 gives a description of the different groups and Fig. 6 shows an example with its segmentation.

The lumen detection has been validated in terms of true localizations (TL), false localizations (FL) and no localizations (NL). We have used Precision, $Prec = \#TL/(\#TL + \#FL)$, and Recall, $Rec = \#TL/(\#TL + \#NL)$, scores to summarize the performance.

4   Experimental Results

The complete methodology has been trained using 30 images per endoscopy type. The optimal parameter values have been chosen to maximize the number

---

[1] http://iam.cvc.uab.es/downloads/

Table 2. Precision and recall results on lumen centre detection.

Type of image	TL	FL	NL	Prec %	Rec %
Bronchoscopy (single lumen) $\#lumen = 76$, $\#nolumen = 10$	76	3	0	96.20	100
Bronchoscopy (multilumen) $\#lumen = 30$	28	0	2	100	93.33
Colononoscopy $\#lumen = 77, \#nolumen = 18$	75	4	2	94.94	97.40

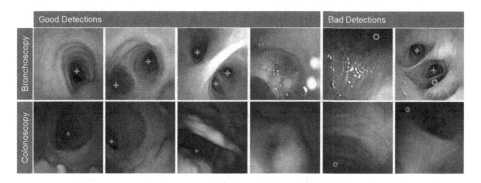

Fig. 7. Qualitative lumen centre detection results. Good detections marked with green crosses and bad ones with green circles. (Color figure online)

of candidate points inside the ground truth. The final values of the different parameters are: DRI $\sigma = 1/24$, $Th_{LK} = 0.12$ for bronchoscopy and $Th_{LK} = 0.14$ for colonoscopy.

Precision and Recall results are given in Table 2. Precision and Recall are over 93 % regardless of the type of image and lumen multiplicity. We only miss 4 lumens: 2 in colonoscopy and 2 in bronchoscopy (all in multi lumen images). We also carried out an experiment to assess the potential of our method to detect lumen presence in the images. It is worth noticing that in the absence of lumen our algorithm does not detect any centre in 8/10 bronchoscopy images and in 16/18 colonoscopy images.

Figure 7 shows qualitative results including good and bad detections. The first 3 columns in the image show examples of good lumen centre detection in single and multi lumen images. Column 4 shows an example of the potential of our method on detecting lumen presence: we can observe that no centre point is marked in the image. The erroneous detections are shown in columns 5 (lumen detection with no lumen presence) and 6. It is worth to mention that in some cases like the ones shown Fig. 7 it is unclear if our algorithm has not really performed well due to the fact that when making a ground truth sometimes there is a great variability on delimiting the lumen region -even the presence/absence of lumen in certain images depend of the experts' criteria-.

All the experiments shown in this section have been performed in a PC with an Intel i7 processor with 16 GB of RAM. The whole processing of one frame takes 0.057 s for bronchoscopy videos and 0.4 s for colonoscopy videos. The difference in computational time is related with the resolution of the image.

5   Conclusions

The detection of the lumen centre is useful for several applications, such as scene description, 3D reconstruction processes or helping in computer aided diagnosis. Moreover, by detecting accurately the lumen centre we can potentially obtain the navigation path inside the organ which could be useful for quality assessment purposes or the following-up of injured tissues. This paper presents a novel lumen centre detection based on a model of appearance and geometry valid for the respiratory and gastrointestinal systems. The presented experimental show a reliable performance on an extensive database that contains images from two modalities (bronchoscopy and colonoscopy) and includes images with multiple lumens and without them.

Acknowledgments. This work was supported by a research grant from Universitat Autónoma de Barcelona 471-01- 2/2010 and by Spanish projects $TIN2009 - 10435$, $TIN2009 - 13618$ and $TIN2012 - 33116$.

References

1. Sucar, L.E., Gillies, D.F.: Knowledge-based assistant for colonscopy. In: Proceedings of the 3rd International Conference on Industrial and Engineering Applications of Artificial Intelligence and Expert Systems, vol. 2, pp. 665–672 (1990)
2. Phee, S., Ng, W., Chen, I., Seow-Choen, F., Davies, B.: Automation of colonoscopy. ii. visual control aspects. Eng. Med. Biol. Mag. IEEE **17**(3), 81–88 (1998)
3. Asari, K.V.: A fast and accurate segmentation technique for the extraction of gastrointestinal lumen from endoscopic images. Med. Eng. Phys. **22**(2), 89–96 (2000)
4. Gallo, G., Torrisi, A.: Lumen detection in endoscopic images: a boosting classification approach. Int. J. Adv. Intell. Syst. **5**(1–2), 127–134 (2012)
5. Zabulis, X., Argyros, A.A., Tsakiris, D.P.: Lumen detection for capsule endoscopy. In: IEEE/RSJ International Conference on Intelligent Robots and Systems, IROS 2008. pp. 3921–3926. IEEE (2008)
6. Masters, I., Eastburn, M., et al.: A new method for objective identification and measurement of airway lumenin paediatric flexible videobronchoscopy. Thorax **60**(8), 652 (2005)
7. McFawn, P., Forkert, L., Fisher, J.: A new method to perform quantitative measurement of bronchoscopic images. ERJ **18**(5), 817–826 (2001)
8. Sanchez, C., Gil, D., Rosell, A., Andaluz, A., Sanchez, F.J.: Segmentation of tracheal rings in videobronchoscopy combining geometry and appearance. In: VISAPP 2013, vol. 1, pp. 153–161 (2013)
9. Bernal, J., Sánchez, J., Vilariño, F.: Impact of image preprocessing methods on polyp localization in colonoscopy frames. In: Proceedings of the 35th International Conference of the IEEE EMBC (Osaka, Japan), July 2013 (in press)
10. Fawcett, T.: An introduction to roc analysis. PR **27**(8), 861–874 (2006)

Automatic Markov Random Field Segmentation of Susceptibility-Weighted MR Venography

Silvain Bériault[(✉)], Marika Archambault-Wallenburg,
Abbas F. Sadikot, D. Louis Collins, and G. Bruce Pike

McConnell Brain Imaging Centre, Montreal Neurological Institute,
3801 University Street, Montreal, QC H3A 2B4, Canada
silvain.beriault@mail.mcgill.ca

Abstract. Patient-specific cerebrovascular modeling provides essential information to facilitate the identification of vessel-free trajectories in functional neurosurgery. However, standard gadolinium models used clinically are often incomplete due to the extent of manual labor required to segment the vessels and because gadolinium contrast decreases rapidly with vessel size. In this work, we propose an automatic method, based on the Markov Random Field (MRF) theory, to segment venous blood vessels from dense susceptibility-weighted imaging (SWI) venography datasets. Unlike conventional isotropic auto-logistic MRF, our MRF design anisotropically favors the neighboring influence of voxels classified as "vessels" to better preserve thin vessels imaged by SWI. Results show that MRF segmentation of deep veins compares well with standard scale-space vesselness analysis. Most importantly, we demonstrate automatic segmentation of superficial veins on SWI and creation of denser 3D vascular models that may improve clinical gadolinium-based models.

Keywords: MR venography · Susceptibility-weighted imaging · Markov random fields · Image-guided neurosurgery · Deep brain stimulation

1 Introduction

With a reported incidence rate as high as 5 % in recent literature [1], hemorrhagic complications pose a high risk of devastating post-operative neurological deficits in functional image-guided neurosurgery. During the pre-surgical planning stage, patient-specific 3D models of the cerebral vasculature are commonly created to guide the neurosurgeon in identifying vessel-free insertion trajectories. In many centers, this task consists of segmenting the cerebral vasculature, either manually or semi-automatically, from a gadolinium-enhanced T1w MRI dataset. However, these models are often incomplete due to the extent of manual labor required and because gadolinium enhancement decreases rapidly in smaller vessels. This work describes a new framework for the automatic segmentation of susceptibility-weighed imaging (SWI) venography datasets.

M. Erdt et al. (Eds.): CLIP 2013, LNCS 8361, pp. 39–47, 2014.
DOI: 10.1007/978-3-319-05666-1_6, © Springer International Publishing Switzerland 2014

Susceptibility weighted imaging (SWI) [2] is a relatively new T2*-weighted gradient echo MRI technique that exploits both the magnitude and phase of the complex MRI signal to increase sensitivity to deoxygenated (venous) blood and to deep brain structures rich in iron content. SWI already provides useful information in a variety of clinical applications including traumatic brain injury, vascular malformations, strokes and neurodegenerative disorders [3]. However, for neurosurgical planning purposes, the reversed vessel contrast imaged by SWI poses new segmentation challenges.

Although several automatic vessel segmentation methods have been proposed in the computer-vision literature [4], techniques that were successfully applied to SWI most often fall under the categories of scale-space analysis or statistical models [5]. Multi-scale "vesselness" filtering methods [6, 7] were shown to produce acceptable results on SWI for deep veins [5, 8], but not for superficial veins [9]. This is due to the absence of a fully defined "tubular-like" 3D contrast between surface veins and surrounding skull. However, surface vein avoidance is essential in functional neurosurgery [10]. Alternatively, statistical methods using local intensity thresholds were investigated [5] but they tend to necessitate post-processing to improve the results.

This paper presents a new statistical segmentation framework based on the Markov Random Field (MRF) theory, and extends the previous work of Hassouna *et al.* [11] originally applied to time-of-flight (TOF) angiography. MRFs are a key step in many segmentation applications to incorporate spatial dependencies among neighboring voxels. For simplicity, the influence of neighboring voxels is often considered isotropic. While this assumption holds for blob-like regions and may hold for the segmentation of major arteries imaged by TOF, an isotropic assumption does not suffice for preserving thinner vessels imaged by SWI. In this work, we describe the implementation of an anisotropic MRF with spatially varying neighborhood influence.

2 Methods

SWI segmentation is implemented as a labeling problem. Each site in the dataset (i.e. the voxels) is labeled as either vessel (V) or tissue (T). Let $S = \{1, \ldots, N\}$ denote the sites and $L = \{V, T\}$ the possible labels. Let $Y = \{y_1, \ldots y_2, \ldots, y_N\}$, $X = \{x_1, \ldots x_2, \ldots, x_N\}$ denote respectively the observed voxel intensity and the output classification at each site in S. The segmentation is performed in three steps:

1. An initial labeling X is found based on the observed intensities Y by expectation maximization (EM).
2. This initial segmentation is further refined with an auto-logistic MRF model to integrate spatial dependencies about the classification of neighboring sites.
3. A skull stripping procedure is computed to distinguish between surface veins and dark-appearing skull.

2.1 Statistical Model

Vessel and brain tissue classes are modeled as a mixture of two normal distributions with parameters $\theta_l = \{w_l, u_l, \sigma_l^2\}$, $l \in \{V, T\}$, where w_l represents the proportions between the two classes. An EM algorithm is applied iteratively for finding the maximum-likelihood estimate of the parameters $\theta_v = \{w_v, u_v, \sigma_v^2\}$ and $\theta_T = \{w_T, u_T, \sigma_T^2\}$. During the E step, the model parameters $\{\theta_v, \theta_T\}$ are held fixed and the posterior probability $f^k(l|y_i)$ of voxel i belonging to class l given its intensity y_i is calculated. During the M step, the model parameters $\{\theta_v, \theta_T\}$ are updated for the next iteration $(k + 1)$. The EM algorithm is applied to brain voxels only (an approximate brain mask is estimated using a co-registered T1w dataset). Proportions w_v^0 and w_T^0 are initialized to 0.05 and 0.95 since blood vessels occupy less than 5 % of the whole brain volume. A simple Otsu threshold is sufficient to estimate initial $\{\mu_l^0, \sigma_l^0\}$ values for the V and T classes. Upon EM convergence, the labeling X for all sites in S is assigned to maximize $f(l|y_i)$:

$$x_i = \arg \max_{l \in \{V, T\}} f(l|y_i), \forall i \in S, \tag{1}$$

$$\text{with } f(l|y_i) = \frac{w_l f(y_i|l)}{\sum_{j=1}^{L} w_j f(y_i|l)}, \text{ and } f(y_i|l) = \left(\frac{1}{\sqrt{2\pi\sigma_l^2}}\right) \exp\left(\frac{-(y_i - \mu_l)^2}{\sqrt{2\sigma_l^2}}\right). \tag{2}$$

2.2 Anisotropic Auto-logistic MRF Model

We implemented an auto-logistic MRF model to refine the initial EM classification by taking into account the classification of neighboring voxels $x_j \in \eta_i$. In our case, η_i is defined to contain all sites x_j within a $3 \times 3 \times 3$ neighborhood of x_i. In the MRF theory, the unknown classification X is modeled as a random process that, according to the Hammersley-Clifford theorem, must obey a Gibbs distribution of the form: $P(X) = Z^{-1}\exp(-U(X))$, where $Z = \sum \exp(-U(X))$ is a normalizing constant called the partition function containing all possible configurations of X. Clearly, exact computation of the partition function on 3D volumetric data is an intractable combinatorial problem. However, it can be avoided if all parameters defining $U(X)$ are properly estimated. In the auto-logistic MRF case, the energy function $U(X)$ is expressed as the sum of clique potential over all possible cliques (a clique is a subset of sites S). When only up to pair-site interactions are considered, the energy function takes the form:

$$U(X) = \sum_{i \in S} \log(f(l|y_i)) + \sum_{i \in S, j \in \eta_i} \beta_{ij} x_i x_j. \tag{3}$$

In (3), the first summation describes the unary association between voxel intensity y_i and class probabilities (see Sect. 2.1). The second summation describes the interaction between classification of voxel x_i and neighboring voxel x_j. β_{ij} is a clique potential parameter that encodes the specific interaction between each voxel pair. Similarity between neighboring voxels is favored when $\beta_{ij} > 0$. In the isotropic case, β_{ij} is either proportional to distance between sites i and j, or constant ($\beta_{ij} = \beta$) to reduce the number of estimated parameters. However, an isotropic MRF configuration applied to SWI will eliminate many thin veins simply because a majority of neighboring voxels would be classified as tissue. Instead, we implemented an anisotropic MRF where potential values β_{ij} are configured to favor the influence of neighboring voxels classified as vessel over those classified as tissue. Since the blood vessels in the dataset do not have the same orientation, the MRF is non-homogeneous, meaning the potential values β_{ij} vary with the spatial location of x_i. Since it is impractical to estimate β_{ij} for all possible voxel pairs in the dataset, we limit the potential β_{ij} to take a constant value of either β_V or β_T such that:

$$\beta_{ij} = \beta_{x_j} = \begin{cases} \beta_V, x_j = V \\ \beta_T, x_j = T \end{cases}. \tag{4}$$

When $\beta_V > \beta_T$, it takes fewer neighboring voxels x_j classified as V, within the local neighborhood η_i, to change the classification of voxel x_i from T to V then in the isotropic case. Reciprocally, it takes more voxels x_j classified as T to change the classification of voxel x_i from V to T then in the isotropic case. The relationship between β_V and β_T was estimated using the maximum pseudo-likelihood (PL) estimation method: $PL(X) = \prod_{x_i \in S} P(x_i | x_{\eta_i})$, with

$$P(x_i | x_{\eta_i}) = \frac{\exp\left(\sum_{j \in \eta_i} \beta_{x_j} x_i x_j\right)}{1 + \exp\left(\sum_{j \in \eta_i} \beta_{x_j} x_j\right)}. \tag{5}$$

Thus a ratio β_V / β_T of 3.45 was estimated and used. With β_V and β_T terms described, the MRF is then solved using the iterated conditional mode method (ICM).

2.3   Surface Veins Extraction

Intensity-based classification does not permit separation between surface veins and skull, both labeled as V due to their similar intensities. As a final step, we model surface vasculature as concavities within the tissue surface. A skull-stripping mask that preserves brain tissue and surface veins is first computed via a binary majority filter applied iteratively to the T class. This filter approximates the convex hull of the T class. Then, vessel concavities are detected using a modified ball filter [12] that measures the local widening within a large neighborhood R_i for all surface voxels x_i classified as V.

$$E_R(i) = E_R'(i) + x_j \sum_{j \in R_i} E_R'(j), \text{ with } E_R'(i) = \sum_{j \in R_i} \chi(x_j), \chi(x_j) = \begin{cases} 0 x_j = T \\ 1 x_j = V \end{cases}. \tag{6}$$

Vessel concavities are detected by computing the ball measure twice, once with $R_i = sphere$ (a standard sphere shape centered at x_i) and once with $R_i = sheet$ (a local 3D sheet-like shape of the brain surface also centered at x_i), to verify that $E_{R = ball}(i) \gg E_{R = sheet}(i)$.

3   Results and Discussion

SWI acquisitions were performed on a 3T Siemens TIM Trio scanner with a 32-channel head coil and we used a multi-echo acquisition strategy to increase signal-to-noise ratio [13]. Thus, magnitude and phase datasets were acquired from a 3D gradient echo sequence with transverse orientation, $0.5 \times 0.5 \times 1$-mm resolution, 5 equally spaced echo times (TE) within the range 13–41 ms, a repetition time (TR) of 48 ms and a flip angle (α) of 17° for a total acquisition time of 10:24 min using GRAPPA acceleration (factor of 2). The first echo is fully flow compensated. The third and fifth echoes are flow compensated in the readout direction. Magnitude and phase images from each echo are combined by standard SWI reconstruction [2]. SWI reconstructed images are then averaged. The average dataset is resampled to 0.5-mm isotropic resolution, denoised with a non local means algorithm [14] and corrected for intensity non-uniformity [15].

3.1   Qualitative Evaluation

An example of MRF-based SWI segmentation is illustrated in Fig. 1. Figure 1a shows a 10-mm minimum intensity projection (mIP) slab of raw SWI data taken at the level of the lateral ventricles (deep venous system). Figure 1b show the MRF segmentation output and Fig. 1c shows the output of conventional multi-scale vesselness filtering using Frangi et al.'s [6] method with typical parameters: $\sigma = [0.5$–$2.5]$, $\Delta\sigma = 0.25$; $\alpha = 0.5$, $\beta = 0.5$, $\gamma = $ half the maximal Hessian norm. MRF segmentation provides a good fit to the raw SWI data, even for smaller lower-contrast septal and subependymal veins, and compares well with the vesselness output. Good agreement between the two vessel extraction techniques is observed up to voxels with very low vesselness value.

The key advantage of MRF segmentation over conventional vesselness filtering is illustrated in Fig. 2. Figure 2a shows a single SWI slice taken at the brain surface level. Figure 2b, c respectively show the output of EM (Sect. 2.1) and MRF/skull-stripping

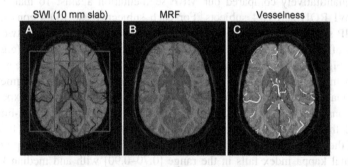

Fig. 1. Illustrative example of MRF-based segmentation at the level of the lateral ventricles. **(a)** A 10-mm minimum intensity projection (minIP) transverse slab from a raw SWI dataset **(b)** MRF segmentation. **(c)** Comparison to scale-space vesselness filtering. **(red boxes)** ROIs of the deep venous system and left/right sub-cortical veins used for validation of Sect. 3.2. (Color figure online)

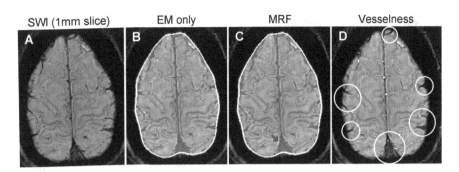

Fig. 2. Automatic segmentation of the surface vasculature. (a) A raw SWI slice at native resolution. (b) Output of EM segmentation. (c) Output of MRF segmentation and skull stripping (white contour) (d) Comparison with scale-space vesselness filtering. Vesselness filtering does not segment the SSS and the superficial cerebral veins (see white circles). (**blue arrow**) MRF regularization of SSS (**Green arrows**) Examples of thin, transversely oriented, vessels preserved during the MRF stage. (Color figure online)

(Sects. 2.2 and 2.3), in comparison to vesselness segmentation (Fig. 2d). At the brain surface, the MRF method achieves proper segmentation of the superior sagittal sinus (SSS) and of smaller superficial vessels. These vessels are not detected by vesselness filtering (see white circles) because they do not fit the tubular assumption. Furthermore, the SSS is particularly challenging to segment on SWI because of the lower contrast. Consequently, after the EM stage, several voxels belonging to the SSS are misclassified as "tissue". The integration of spatial dependencies (MRF stage) improves the SSS segmentation (see blue arrow). This regularization is achieved without eliminating thin, transversely oriented, vessels (see green arrows).

3.2   Quantitative Evaluation

We also quantitatively compared our MRF segmentation against 16 manually segmented SWI ROIs across 4 subjects. For each subject, these ROIs consist of one 10-mm mIP slab of the deep venous system (medial region of Fig. 1a), two 10-mm mIP slabs of the sub-cortical veins on the left and right hemispheres (e.g. lateral regions of Fig. 1a) and one whole slice taken at the brain surface level (e.g. Fig. 2). The kappa index was computed between the MRF and expert-based segmentations (MRF-manual kappa), and between conventional vesselness (v) and expert-based segmentations (v-manual kappa). Since the vesselness segmentation is non-binary, we considered the maximal v-manual kappa index on a range of possible thresholds. Results of the comparison are shown in Table 1. For sub-cortical and deep veins, the MRF-manual kappa index falls in the range [0.70–0.90] with and median kappa of 0.86. Furthermore, the MRF-manual is higher then the maximal v-manual kappa index for 11 out of 12 slabs. At brain surface, the maximal v-manual kappa index drops to the range [0.36–0.56] while the MRF-manual kappa index stays in the range [0.77–0.84].

Table 1. Comparison between MRF-manual and maximal (υ)esselness-manual kappa indexes for 16 ROIs accross four subjects.

ROI	Subject 1		Subject 2		Subject 3		Subject 4	
	MRF	υ	MRF	υ	MRF	υ	MRF	υ
Deep venous system	0.85	0.76	0.85	0.79	0.83	0.76	0.80	0.77
Left subcortical veins	0.87	0.82	0.70	0.81	0.89	0.74	0.88	0.80
Right subcortical veins	0.90	0.81	0.86	0.79	0.86	0.78	0.86	0.81
Surface veins	**0.80**	**0.48**	**0.84**	**0.36**	**0.77**	**0.51**	**0.82**	**0.56**

3.3 Application to Neurosurgical Planning

As stated in introduction, patient-specific 3D models of the cerebral vasculature (and surface vasculature in particular) are often used to identify vessel-free insertion trajectories in minimally invasive functional neurosurgery. Figure 3 shows some examples of cerebrovascular models created from SWI and Gadolinium-enhanced MRI. Four patients who underwent deep brain stimulation (DBS) surgery were scanned with both MRI protocols. The SWI datasets (top row) were segmented using the automatic MRF method. The gadolinium-enhanced datasets (bottom row) were manually segmented on the Medtronic StealthStation® platform by the clinical neuronavigation team and used for planning the actual DBS intervention. The manually processed clinical models may qualitatively appear smoother but are limited to the main vasculature only and the clinical model for subject 4 is particularly incomplete. Automatically processed SWI datasets result in denser models of the surface veins and more side branches can be observed.

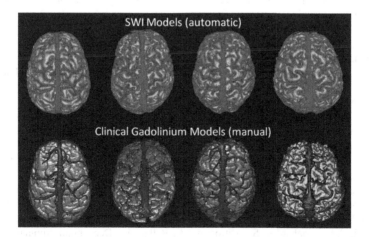

Fig. 3 (top row) Automatic reconstruction of surface veins by MRF on SWI. (bottom row) Comparison to manual segmentation on gadolinium enhanced MRI, created using the Medtronic StealthStation® platform, and used clinically for DBS planning.

4 Conclusion

Avoiding the cerebral vasculature is essential in functional neurosurgery to minimize risks of post-operative neurological deficits. Due to the high inter-subject variability, the cerebral vasculature must be imaged and segmented for each patient individually. For this purpose, SWI provides more detailed imaging of cerebral veins in comparison to conventional gadolinium protocols without requiring injection of contrast agent. However, automatic segmentation of SWI vasculature is challenging, especially at brain surface, due to the reversed venous contrast. In this work, we presented an anisotropic MRF framework to segment both sub-cortical and the surface vasculature on SWI data. To our knowledge, this is the first method that applies MRF for SWI segmentation and, most importantly, to demonstrate adequate SWI segmentation of the surface vasculature. Future work will concentrate on extending this MRF approach for segmenting SWI veins at the basal ganglia level and distinguishing them from other hypo-intense (iron-rich) nuclei present in this area.

References

1. Zrinzo, L., Foltynie, T., Limousin, P., Hariz, M.I.: Reducing hemorrhagic complications in functional neurosurgery: a large case series and systematic literature review. J. Neurosurg. **116**, 84–94 (2012)
2. Haacke, E.M., Xu, Y., Cheng, Y.C., Reichenbach, J.R.: Susceptibility weighted imaging (SWI). Magn. Reson. Med. **52**, 612–618 (2004)
3. Mittal, S., Wu, Z., Neelavalli, J., Haacke, E.M.: Susceptibility-weighted imaging: technical aspects and clinical applications, part 2. AJNR Am. J. Neuroradiol. **30**, 232–252 (2009)
4. Lesage, D., Angelini, E.D., Bloch, I., Funka-Lea, G.: A review of 3D vessel lumen segmentation techniques: models, features and extraction schemes. Med. Image Anal. **13**, 819–845 (2009)
5. Haacke, E.M., Reichenbach, J.R.: Susceptibility weighted imaging in MRI: basic concepts and clinical applications. Wiley-Blackwell, Hoboken (2011)
6. Frangi, A., Niessen, W., Vincken, K., Viergever, M.: Multiscale vessel enhancement filtering. In: Wells, W.M., Colchester, A.C.F., Delp, S.L. (eds.) MICCAI 1998. LNCS, vol. 1496, pp. 130–137. Springer, Heidelberg (1998)
7. Manniesing, R., Viergever, M.A., Niessen, W.J.: Vessel enhancing diffusion: a scale space representation of vessel structures. Med. Image Anal. **10**, 815–825 (2006)
8. Koopmans, P.J., Manniesing, R., Niessen, W.J., Viergever, M.A., Barth, M.: MR venography of the human brain using susceptibility weighted imaging at very high field strength. MAGMA **21**, 149–158 (2008)
9. Beriault, S., Subaie, F.A., Collins, D.L., Sadikot, A.F., Pike, G.B.: A multi-modal approach to computer-assisted deep brain stimulation trajectory planning. Int. J. Comput. Assist. Radiol. Surg. **7**, 687–704 (2012)
10. Benabid, A.L., Chabardes, S., Mitrofanis, J., Pollak, P.: Deep brain stimulation of the subthalamic nucleus for the treatment of Parkinson's disease. Lancet Neurol. **8**, 67–81 (2009)
11. Hassouna, M.S., Farag, A.A., Hushek, S., Moriarty, T.: Cerebrovascular segmentation from TOF using stochastic models. Med. Image Anal. **10**, 2–18 (2006)

12. Nain, D., Yezzi, A., Turk, G.: Vessel segmentation using a shape driven flow. In: Barillot, C., Haynor, D.R., Hellier, P. (eds.) MICCAI 2004. LNCS, vol. 3216, pp. 51–59. Springer, Heidelberg (2004)

13. Denk, C., Rauscher, A.: Susceptibility weighted imaging with multiple echoes. J. Magn. Reson. Imag. **31**, 185–191 (2010)

14. Coupe, P., Yger, P., Prima, S., Hellier, P., Kervrann, C., Barillot, C.: An optimized blockwise nonlocal means denoising filter for 3-D magnetic resonance images. IEEE Trans. Med. Imag. **27**, 425–441 (2008)

15. Sled, J.G., Zijdenbos, A.P., Evans, A.C.: A nonparametric method for automatic correction of intensity nonuniformity in MRI data. IEEE Trans. Med. Imag. **17**, 87–97 (1998)

MR Enterography Image Fusion in Small Bowel Analysis

Juan J. Cerrolaza$^{(\boxtimes)}$, Nabile M. Safdar, Raymond W. Sze,
and Marius George Linguraru

Sheikh Zayed Institute for Pediatric Surgical Innovation,
Children's National Medical Center, Washington, DC, USA
{jcerrola,nsafdar,rsze,mlingura}@childrensnational.org

Abstract. In the last years, the use of magnetic resonance enterography to evaluate inflammatory bowel diseases has become a mainstay, thanks to its non-ionizing nature, and to the advent of faster sequences that are less sensitive to motion artifacts. In this work we present a novel multimodal image merging framework able to combine the detailed structural information, and the small bowel motility provided by the SSFSE and the FIESTA sequence, respectively. Once the breathing motion has been eliminated via non-rigid B-spline based registration, we create a personalized peristaltic activity map from the FIESTA sequence using optical flow analysis. Defining a new multimodal similarity measure, the two nearest sets of FIESTA frames are projected over the SSFSE slices, leading to a new image that provides specific structural and functional information of the patient simultaneously. The practical utility of these new images has been successfully evaluated in a preliminary study with 13 cases, showing its potential for planning small bowel interventions, and patients' diagnosis and follow up.

Keywords: Small bowel · Crohn's disease · MR enterography · SSFSE · FIESTA · Optical flow · Multimodal similarity

1 Introduction

According to recent studies, there has been an increase in the incidence of inflammatory bowel diseases at a global level [1]. In particular, Crohn's disease affects between 3.1 and 14.6 cases per 100,000 person-years in North America. The disease typically manifests in the lower part of the small bowel and the colon, with the former involved in the 80 % of the diagnosed cases. While traditional colonoscopy allows access and diagnosis to the colon, the small bowel is especially difficult to diagnose due to poor access and complex anatomy [3]. Thanks to advances in the field of diagnostic imaging, the interest in small bowel imaging has increased in the last years and new techniques were introduced, not only in the diagnosis, but also to guide the treatment of patients with established Crohn's disease. These technological advances have led to the

M. Erdt et al. (Eds.): CLIP 2013, LNCS 8361, pp. 48–56, 2014.
DOI: 10.1007/978-3-319-05666-1_7, © Springer International Publishing Switzerland 2014

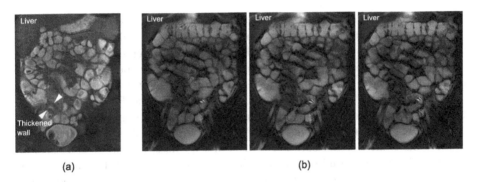

Fig. 1. MRE data. (a) Example of a case diagnosed with Crohn's disease. The SSFSE image allows to appreciate the wall thickness in the terminal ileum. (b) Three different frames of a FIESTA sequence showing the peristalsis of the small bowel (see the segments pointed by the colored arrows). For clarity, images in (b) don't show respiratory motion.

development and clinical implementation of optimized MR imaging protocols, where magnetic resonance enterography (MRE) has become a mainstay in the evaluation of small bowel disease. Its non-invasive nature, and the absence of ionizing radiation, make it especially useful in the pediatric population and for patients who require serial imaging [2]. High resolution ultra-fast sequences are particularly suitable in the study of the small bowel by MRE, providing sharp images of the anatomy of the intestine. Fast Imaging Employing Steady-State Acquisition (FIESTA) sequence is a free-breathing sequence in which a single volume of the abdomen is continuously imaged over a period of seconds to allow monitoring and quantifying the small bowel peristalsis (Fig. 1(b)). Though the use of this cine sequence improves lesion detection, the presence of black boundary artifacts along the bowel wall may mask small lesions or abnormalities. This problem does not occur in the Single-Shot Fast Spin Echo (SSFSE) sequence, an ultrafast sequence that enables to acquire whole MR data in a single radio frequency excitation. This static image allows to identify areas with increased mural thickness (Fig. 1(a)), frequently associated with bowel sections affected by Crohn's disease.

To the best of our knowledge, very few works in the field of medical image processing have tried to address the characterization or modeling of the small intestine. Holmes et al. [3] present an interactive region growing based segmentation framework of the small bowel area for MRE imaging. However, the inherent problems associated with the intestine make it difficult to extract conclusive topological information from the set of voxels obtained (location of small bowel), which limits its practical applicability. Alternatively, Zhang et al. [4] segmented the small bowel from high resolution contrast-enhanced CT images using information from the surrounding mesenteric arterial vasculature; however, the technique is based on images acquired under high radiation.

From a completely different perspective, this work presents a new tool for the diagnosis, treatment, and follow up of patients with Crohn's disease. By merging the information provided by the two MRE sequences presented above (FIESTA and SSFSE), we create a new set of images that allows the specialist to simultaneously analyze the patient's structural details provided by the SSFSE sequence, and the particular peristaltic activity extracted from the FIESTA sequence. First, we create a personalized intestinal peristaltic activity maps of the patient from the FIESTA set of frames by means of the optical flow field. Defining a multimodal similarity measure between both sequences, the two nearest sets of FIESTA frames are combined to obtain the estimated peristaltic activity for every SSFSE image. The multi-sequence information is then combined via multimodal image registration.

2   Methods

2.1   Breathing Compensation and Peristalsis Map

In the study of the small bowel, the FIESTA sequence is used to create a coronal cine sequence of images that reflects the temporal evolution of the area, i.e., monitoring the small bowel peristaltic motion. As image acquisition is relatively slow (>100 s. per sequence), both respiratory and peristaltic motions are present in these images. Since the clinical interest is only the peristalsis, the respiratory component must be corrected.

Let $\{\mathbf{X}_{i,t}\}$, represents the set of frames of the FIESTA sequence acquired at position $i = 1, \ldots, N$ over time $t = 1, \cdots, T$ (i.e., i defines the location in the sagittal axis in which the coronal images are acquired), where the time instants t have been discretized for simplicity of notation. The effects of the respiratory cycle can be graphically observed by concatenating the horizontal intensity projection of each frame, $[\mathbf{x}_{i,1}, \ldots, \mathbf{x}_{i,T}]$, where T is the number of frames (Fig. 2(a)). Though the main effect of the respiratory cycle is a vertical displacement of the abdominal organs in the FIESTA sequence, its effects cannot be accurately compensated by means of simple rigid registration. Instead, we perform a non-rigid linear B-spline based registration over each $i - th$ set of frames, using a least-square cost function, and the $t_{ref} - th$ frame, $\mathbf{X}_{i,t_{ref}}$, as reference (Fig. 2(b)). In particular, $t_{ref} - th$ is a frame in the middle of the breathing cycle (Fig. 2(c)-(e)). The use of first order B-splines allows us to compensate these respiratory effects that affect the entire abdomen without introducing spurious local deformations that could alter the actual peristalsis.

Suppose now $\left\{\widehat{\mathbf{X}}_{i,t}\right\}$ represents the set of registered frames using $\mathbf{X}_{i,t_{ref}}$ as a reference. Once the breathing motion has been compensated, we extract the remaining pattern of apparent motion (i.e., the peristalsis of the small bowel) from this sequence of ordered images. Optical flow theory allows us to model these deformations in the small bowel as flow patterns, that is a vector field whose components, $\mathbf{u}$ and $\mathbf{v}$, represent the local image flow (velocity) at each pixel. In this work we use the widely known differential-based optical flow approach

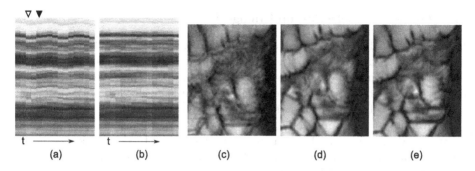

t ⟶   t ⟶

(a)   (b)   (c)   (d)   (e)

Fig. 2. Respiratory motion correction for FIESTA data. (a)(b) Pre- and post-registration horizontal intensity projection over time, respectively. (c) Difference between two frames of the original unregistered sequence (gray regions show where the two frames have the same intensities, while colored areas show where the intensities are different). (d) Registration to a frame at the end of the exhalation phase ($\triangledown$). (e) Registration to a frame in the middle of the respiratory cycle ($\blacktriangledown$). Note that the correction of respiratory motion should not eliminate peristalsis (the residual motion in (e)).

presented by Horn and Schunk [5]. This method uses the typical optical flow constraint equation, imposing an additional global smoothness constraint. Thus, the global energy function to minimize is

$$E = \int \int \left(\nabla \mathbf{X}_{i,t} \cdot \mathbf{V}_i + \frac{\partial \mathbf{X}_{i,t}}{\partial t} \right)^2 + \alpha^2 \left(\|\nabla \mathbf{u}_i\|^2 + \|\nabla \mathbf{v}_i\|^2 \right) dx dy \qquad (1)$$

where $\mathbf{V}_i = [\mathbf{u}_i, \mathbf{v}_i]$ is the optical flow field, and α is the regularization constant. Equation (1) can be minimized by solving the associated Lagrange equation (see [5] for details). Figure 3 illustrates how $\|\mathbf{V}_i\|$ can be used to represent graphically the peristaltic activity of the intestine.

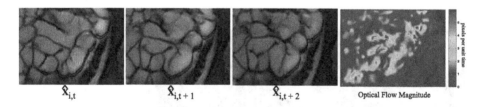

$\hat{\mathbf{X}}_{i,t}$ $\hat{\mathbf{X}}_{i,t+1}$ $\hat{\mathbf{X}}_{i,t+2}$ Optical Flow Magnitude

Fig. 3. Peristalsis motion analysis. Three consecutive registered frames from the FIESTA sequence showing the peristalsis of a particular small bowel section are presented from left. The average optical flow magnitude is shown in the right image and provides a compact graphical representation of the activity in each bowel area.

2.2 Frame Sets Selection and Image Fusion

Before merging the images provided by the SSFSE sequence with the peristaltic activity field extracted from the FIESTA sequence, it is necessary to register both sources of information. Though the MRE protocol could be theoretically configured to acquire both sets of images at the same locations (i.e., at the same positions of the sagittal axis), this is not always possible in practice (i.e., the MRE protocol was not configured with this purpose and thus the spacing between SSFSE and FIESTA images is not the same). In this work, the most general situation is assumed: for each SSFSE image it is necessary to identify the closest sets of FIESTA frames.

Suppose $\mathbf{Y}_j$ represents a SSFSE image acquired at position $j = 1, \ldots, M$, and that $\mathcal{D}(\mathbf{I}_1, \mathbf{I}_2)$ defines a multimodal similarity measure between two images $\mathbf{I}_1$ and $\mathbf{I}_2$. For each $\mathbf{Y}_j$ it is necessary to find the pair of consecutive FIESTA frame sets that maximize $D_{j,i} = E\left[\mathcal{D}\left(\mathbf{Y}_j, \widehat{\mathbf{X}}_{i,t}\right)\right]$. To define the multimodal similarity, $\mathcal{D}(\cdot, \cdot)$, the regularized normalized gradient field (NGF) proposed by Haber and Modersitzki [6] is used. Given an image $\mathbf{I}$, its NGF, $\mathcal{N}(\mathbf{I})$, is defined as $\mathcal{N}(\mathbf{I}) = \nabla \mathbf{I} / \|\nabla \mathbf{I}\|_\varepsilon$. The normalization term is $\|\nabla \mathbf{I}\|_\varepsilon = \left(\sum_{l=1\ldots\ell} \nabla \mathbf{I}_l^2 + \varepsilon^2\right)^{1/2}$, where $\ell = 2$ for $2D$ images, and ε is a measure for boundary jumps (i.e., locations with a high gradient) which can be defined as $\varepsilon = \int |\nabla \mathbf{I}|$. Given a certain point in the image domain, $\mathbf{p} = (x, y)$, the vectors $\mathcal{N}(\mathbf{Y}_j)_{(x,y)}$ and $\mathcal{N}(\mathbf{X}_i)_{(x,y)}$ form an angle $\theta(\mathbf{p})$. Since the gradient fields are normalized, the inner product of the vectors is related to the cosine of this angle, i.e., the higher the inner product, the higher the similarity between both locations. Thus, we can define the global similarity measure between $\mathbf{Y}_j$ and $\mathbf{X}_{i,t}$ as

$$\mathcal{D}\left(\mathbf{Y}_j, \widehat{\mathbf{X}}_{i,t}\right) = E\left[\langle \mathcal{N}(\mathbf{Y}_j), \mathcal{N}(\widehat{\mathbf{X}}_{i,t})\rangle^2\right] = E\left[\mathbf{W}_{j,i,t}(\mathbf{p})^2\right] \tag{2}$$

where $\langle \cdot, \cdot \rangle$, and $\mathbf{W}_{i,j,t}$, represents the inner product operator, and the similarity matrix between both images, respectively. Figure 4 illustrates the FIESTA set selection for a particular SSFSE image.

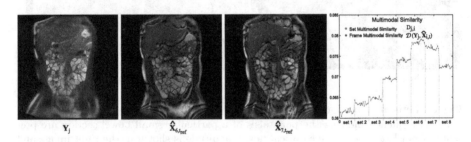

Fig. 4. Multi-sequence MRE fusion. From left we present an example of a SSFSE image, $\mathbf{Y}_j$, and the two closest FIESTA frame sets, $\left\{\widehat{\mathbf{X}}_{6,t}\right\}$, and $\left\{\widehat{\mathbf{X}}_{7,t}\right\}$. The graph on the right shows the multimodal similarity between $\mathbf{Y}_j$ and each FIESTA frame.

Once the corresponding sets of FIESTA frames have been defined, it is possible to estimate the peristaltic activity field for $\mathbf{Y}_j$, PAF_j, as a weighted sum of $\|\mathbf{V}_i\|$ and $\|\mathbf{V}_{i+1}\|$. Suppose $\widehat{\mathbf{Y}}_{j,i}$ is the registered version of $\mathbf{Y}_j$ obtained via multimodal registration to $\mathbf{X}_{i,t_{ref}}$. Assuming that the reference frame belongs to the same phase of the respiratory cycle (see Sect. 2.1), we can approximate $\widehat{\mathbf{Y}}_{j,i} \sim \widehat{\mathbf{Y}}_{j,i+1}$. Thus, PAF_j can be defined as

$$PAF_j = \frac{\widehat{\mathbf{W}}_{j,i} \cdot \|\mathbf{V}_i\| + \widehat{\mathbf{W}}_{j,i+1} \cdot \|\mathbf{V}_{i+1}\|}{\widehat{\mathbf{W}}_{j,i} + \widehat{\mathbf{W}}_{j,i+1}} \tag{3}$$

where $\widehat{\mathbf{W}}_{j,i} = \frac{1}{T}\sum_t \widehat{\mathbf{W}}_{j,i,t}$, and $\widehat{\mathbf{W}}_{j,i,t} = \langle \mathcal{N}\left(\widehat{\mathbf{Y}}_j\right), \mathcal{N}\left(\widehat{\mathbf{X}}_{i,t}\right) \rangle$.

3   Results

The utility of this new MRE-image merging framework was evaluated in 13 studies: 7 healthy cases with no evidence of inflammatory bowel disease, and 6 cases in which the experts detected intestinal pathology. The scans were obtained using two systems, an Optima MR450 1.5T MR GE system, and a Discovery MR750 3.0T MR GE device, which provided 512×512 pixels images with resolutions from 0.82 to 0.94 mm per pixel. The FIESTA sequences were composed by 18 locations/slices with 15 frames per location, and a slice thickness of 8 mm. The SSFSE sequences were formed by 30 slices with one frame per location and 6 mm slice thickness. A new set of images was generated according to the image fusion method described in Sect. 2 ($\alpha = 0.5$). These images were evaluated by an expert radiologist to assess their potential for the diagnosis of inflammatory bowel disease, treatment, and patient follow up. In particular, the expert is presented a map of the bowel motility that identifies an highlights the regions with reduced motility that require attention (structural analysis).

Figures 5(a) and (b) show the SSFSE-FIESTA fusion images of two healthy patients. Though the peristaltic activity seems to be normal, some areas with reduced motility (< 0.5 mm/s) can be appreciated. However, the subsequent structural analysis of these areas did not reveal any evidence of small bowel abnormality. Figure 5(c) shows the SSFSE-FIESTA fusion image of a patient diagnosed with Crohn's disease, whose terminal ileum exhibits a markedly reduced peristalsis (0.4 mm/s). In the case depicted in Fig. 5(d) and (e) there is no sign of thickened walls and most of the small bowel seems to move normally (≥ 0.8 mm/s). However, the last 5 cm of the ileum is narrowed with a proximally dilated bowel, indicative of a possible bowel stricture. The images also indicate correctly how the reduced motility of the involved areas (marked with arrow in the image). The case depicted in Fig. 5(e) belongs to the same patient shown in Fig. 1(a). Using the new combined image, it is possible to observe simultaneously the wall thickness of the localized segment of the bowel (from SSFSE), and the reduced motility of this area (from the analysis of FIESTA), below 0.6 mm/s. These findings are indicative imaging biomarkers of Crohn's disease.

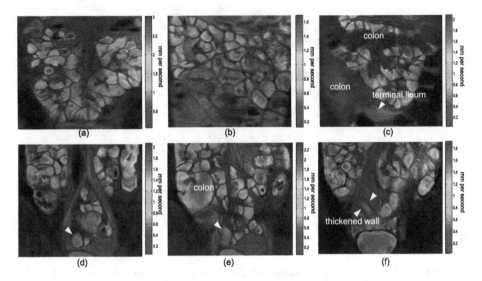

Fig. 5. SSFSE-FIESTA fusion images. (a)(b) Fusion images of two healthy patients. (c) Patient with reduced peristalsis localized in the terminal ileum. (d,e) Different slices of the same patient. The terminal ileum is narrowed with proximal dilatation (marked with arrows). (d) Patient with significant bowel wall thickening (marked with arrows) and reduced motility.

We quantified that healthy small bowel motility can go up to $3\,mm/s$, while in the areas of reduced motility the motion of the bowel was less than $0.6\,mm/s$. However, the inter- and intraindividual variability of small bowel motility [7] must be considered when abnormalities are being sought.

Merging SSFSE and the FIESTA sequences, in combination with the quantitative analysis of small bowel motility, offers a new tool for diagnosis and personalized treatment planning of intestinal diseases. These new images allow to simultaneously study the structural information along with the peristaltic activity in a single image, making it easier and faster to identify problematic areas that require clinical attention. The peristaltic activity map created is also very useful in patient follow up, such as response to treatment, allowing the quantitative comparison of the motility of specific areas of the small bowel in different studies of the same patient.

4   Conclusion

It is critical for gastroenterologists managing patients with inflammatory bowel disease to accurately identify affected areas of small bowel and to monitor disease progression as they adjust their therapy over time. Worsening of small bowel disease will prompt escalation of medical therapy. In severe cases, portions of the bowel may have to be resected surgically and accurate localization of the abnormal small bowel may come largely from MR enterography. Because the implications for treatment and prognosis are high, the ability to better identify and visualize areas of abnormal bowel motility may improve detection and have significant implications for treatment decisions. A combination of FIESTA and the SSFSE sequences is particularly essential in this context. While the former provides information about the motility, the second reveals structural details, like the thickness of the bowel wall. Merging the information from both sequences, the new framework presented in this work allows to create a new set of images of clinical utility for the fast and accurate assessment of inflammatory bowel diseases. Once the respiratory movement in the FIESTA sequence has been eliminated, a peristaltic activity map is generated via optical flow analysis. The projection of these activity maps on the SSFSE images gives rise to a new set of images that provides personalized structural and functional information of the patient simultaneously.

In cases where there are only subtle changes from one MR enterography to the next, the ability to quantify and localize abnormal areas of motility may serve as an important new tool for radiologists when communicating disease burden to their gastroenterology and surgery colleagues. Currently, the lack of visualization or quantification of such abnormal areas leads to high interobserver variability in the interpretation of small bowel disease on MR enterography. A preliminary study with 13 cases revealed the practical utility of these new data in real clinical studies, and their potential for patients' diagnosis and follow up. In the future work, we will develop an automated structural analysis of the bowel and define quantitative measures of inflammatory bowel disease from our new imaging biomarkers. We hypothesize that the improved visualization of abnormal motility in small bowel will improve detection of such areas and reduced interobserver variability. Further evaluation of these techniques will be necessary to determine their ability to affect clinical outcomes.

References

1. Molodecky, N.A., Soon, I.S., et al.: Increasing incidence and prevalence of the inflammatory bowel diseases with time based on systematic review. Gastroenterology **142**(1), 46–54 (2011)
2. Gee, M.S., Nimkin, K., et al.: Prospective evaluation of MR enterography as the primary imaging modality for pediatric crohn disease assessment. Am. J. Roentgenoloy. **197**(1), 224–231 (2011)
3. Holmes, D., Huprich, J., Fidler, J., Robb, R., Fletcher, J.: Feasibility of developing interactive small bowel segmentation from MR enterography. In: Proceedings of MICCAI 2010 Workshop Virtual Colonoscopy and Abdominal Imaging, pp. 105–110 (2010)
4. Zhang, W., Liu, J., et al.: Mesenteric vasculature-guided small bowel segmentation on high-resolution 3D CT angiography scans. In: 9th IEEE International Symposium on Biomedical Imaging (ISBI), pp. 1280–1283 (2012)
5. Horn, B.K.P., Schunk, B.G.: Determining optical flow. Artif. Intell. **17**, 185–203 (1981)

6. Haber, E., Modersitzki, J.: Beyond mutual information: a simple and robust alternative. In: Meinzer, H.-P., Handels, H., Horsch, A., Tolxdorff, T. (eds.) Bildverarbeitung fur die Medizin 2005. Informatik Aktuell, pp. 350–354. Springer, Heidelberg (2005)
7. Kerlin, P., Phillips, S.: Variability of motility of the ileum and jejunum in healthy humans. Gastroenterology **82**, 694–700 (1982)

Landmark-Based Surgical Navigation

Adrian Schneider$^{(\boxtimes)}$, Christian Baumberger, Mathias Griessen, Simon Pezold,
Jörg Beinemann, Philipp Jürgens, and Philippe C. Cattin

Medical Image Analysis Center, University of Basel, Basel, Switzerland
adrian.schneider@unibas.ch

Abstract. Navigational support is a widely adopted technique in surgery
that has become a part of the clinical routine. This navigation support
either comes in the form of an abstract display that shows for example the distance and direction to the target position or in the form of
augmented reality where segmented anatomical structures of interest are
overlaid onto a visual image sequence in real-time.

In this paper we propose a cost-effective real-time augmented reality
approach using an off-the-shelf tablet PC in combination with a novel
2D/3D point correspondence mapping technique. The proposed point
pattern matching algorithm is tailored towards moderate projective distortions and suitable for computational low-power devices. Experiments
and comparisons were done on synthetic images and accuracy was measured on real scenes. The excellent performance is demonstrated by an
Android 3D guidance application for a relevant medical intervention.

Keywords: Augmented reality · Point pattern matching · Navigation

1 Introduction

According to the *World Health Organization*, there are more than one million
surgery-related deaths world-wide per year [12]. One of the reasons is that performing surgical interventions poses very high demands on the spatial sense of
the surgeons. As has been documented by several studies [6,9] intraoperative
3D navigation greatly supports the surgeon in complex interventions and significantly reduces the risk for the patients. However, the currently available systems
for 3D navigation are bulky, complex to operate and expensive.

In this paper, we focus on the development of an image-guided 3D navigation system that can be quickly brought in place, requires minimal training
and is affordable. We show that an off-the-shelf tablet computer can bridge
this gap although certain challenges appear. A common tablet has only one
built-in CMOS camera. Therefore, our 3D navigation system is restricted to
operate in single view mode. Furthermore, a tablet is a computational low-power
environment and thus computationally expensive image processing routines are
inapplicable for real-time applications.

Christian and Adrian contributed equally to this work.

M. Erdt et al. (Eds.): CLIP 2013, LNCS 8361, pp. 57–64, 2014.
DOI: 10.1007/978-3-319-05666-1_8, © Springer International Publishing Switzerland 2014

To increase usability and allow a seamless integration into the surgical work-flow, an intuitive augmented reality (AR) visualization technique is used. In the proposed navigation system, virtual anatomical objects are rendered and superimposed onto the image stream from the camera and shown on the tablet. This requires the determination of the exact 3D position and orientation of the tablet's camera with respect to the patient and handing over these parameters to the virtual camera of the renderer. This brings us to the essential challenge and core contribution of this work, namely the development of an accurate but computationally cheap camera pose estimation.

In applications with only one tracking camera, a reliable camera pose esti-mation method uses 3D/2D point correspondences, where the 2D coordinates represent the pixel locations of detected landmarks and the corresponding 3D coordinates are known with respect to an MR or CT data set of the patient. Hav-ing several of these 3D/2D point correspondences, one can compute the camera pose transformation relative to the 3D coordinate system of the landmarks and therefore render anatomical structures from the right perspective.

Extracting these landmarks from an image has to be efficient and reliable. Fast texture-based methods [4] are prone to perspective distortion [10] and likely to fail on smooth surfaces such as teeth or bone. Therefore we decided to use small, uniformly colored stickers as markers, which can be segmented efficiently by color channel thresholding. In addition, we treat each new image completely separately from the previous frames, i.e. a tracking-by-detection approach was chosen. The advantage of tracking-by-detection is that fast movements do not distract the tracking and there is no accumulation of error or drift over time. The complete segmentation of the landmarks is performed on the GPU of the tablet and results in a binary image. The centers of the circles are then determined by using the blob detector of OpenCV.

Because the proposed landmarks are not accompanied by any unique iden-tifier, such as distinctive colors or unique texture descriptors, there is no direct way to assign the corresponding 3D coordinates to each detected 2D position landmark. What might look like a simple operation at first, turns out to be a challenging task known as *point pattern matching* (PPM) [3]. In our context, a PPM method is required which matches two point patterns (the detected 2D landmarks to the set of known 3D coordinates) related by a projective transfor-mation. Such algorithms exist, but they are computationally too expensive [1] or are restricted to coplanar point patterns [2,3,11]. Optimized SLAM methods [5] might be an option, but their structure-from-motion approach does not match our tracking-by-detection requirement.

A computationally feasible approach is to simplify the problem and match the segmented 2D point set v_S with an initially generated reference 2D point pattern v_R, which is the virtual projection of the 3D landmarks from a *reference direction* (Fig. 1). With that step, projective characteristics are banished from the model but return in the form of projective distortions.

A robust method to handle such distortions is to approximate a complex geo-metric behavior by multiple local low-order transformations [8]. On the basis of

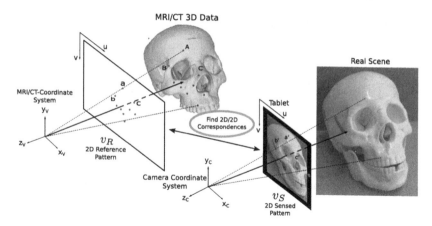

Fig. 1. Simplification of the 3D/2D to a 2D/2D correspondence problem. The blue points denote the 3D object points, the red points the 2D reference pattern projected from the reference direction, and the green points on the tablet the 2D sensed pattern.

this idea, we developed a computationally lightweight algorithm used for rather small point patterns. The newly proposed method is called *Point Recursive Matching* (PRM).

2   Method

The PRM algorithm is based on a recursive structure with an early stopping criterion. Before the algorithm can be applied to find correspondences, point set descriptors Q_R of v_R and Q_S of v_S needs to be computed. The descriptors themselves serve as a look-up table during the recursion and therefore do not need to be recomputed after each iteration. The algorithm is able to handle multiple occlusions since it tries to establish correspondences by locally finding corresponding points and does not try to match the complete pattern at once. By changing the number of nearest point neighbors N_{nb}, among which the solution finding process continues, one can adjust how *locally* the algorithm operates.

Point Set Descriptor. The first step of building the point set descriptor involves the definition of an arbitrarily chosen *base direction*. Subsequently, a descriptor for every point in the point set is computed as follows: compute the connecting vector to every other point in the point set, and compute the angle of this vector with respect to the base direction. The angle of a point to itself is defined as -1. Figure 2 shows two example point descriptors for point a and b. Finally, all the point descriptors are appended in row-direction into a matrix, which forms the complete point set descriptor Q (Fig. 3). Once the two point set descriptors Q_R of v_R and Q_S of v_S are computed, point correspondences can be established with the recursive approach described in the next paragraph.

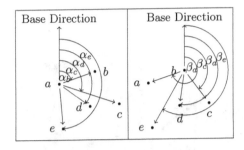

Fig. 2. Two example point descriptors.

Angles					
	a	b	c	d	e
a	-1	α_b	α_c	α_d	α_e
b	β_a	-1	β_c	β_d	β_e
c	γ_a	γ_b	-1	γ_d	γ_e
d	δ_a	δ_b	δ_c	-1	δ_e
e	ϵ_a	ϵ_b	ϵ_c	ϵ_d	-1

Fig. 3. Point set descriptor Q in matrix form.

Matching Algorithm. For practical reasons, we demonstrate the matching algorithm on two example point sets v_R and v_S (Fig. 4, 5, 6 and 7). The set v_S results from the segmentation and therefore has an arbitrary point order. The algorithm starts with the first point of each point set and assumes that these two points correspond to each other. In the example point sets, this corresponds to $a \leftrightarrow a'$ and is shown in Fig. 4.

Next, the algorithm chooses the next point pair among the N_{nb} nearest neighbors of the last assigned correspondence, a respective a'. In this case, the algorithm assigns $b \leftrightarrow b'$ to each other, and reads the angles ϕ_{ab} and $\phi_{a'b'}$ from the pre-computed point set descriptors Q_R and Q_S. In particular these correspond to the entries α_b (Fig. 3) in both Q_R and Q_S. This step is shown in Fig. 5.

The difference of these two angles is kept as the offset between the two point sets $\phi_{offset} = \phi_{ab} - \phi_{a'b'}$. This offset is subtracted in the following from every angle in the sensed point set descriptor Q_S, in order to make it rotation invariant.

The third corresponding point pair is chosen among the not yet assigned N_{nb} nearest neighbor points of b and b', for example the point pair $c \leftrightarrow c'$ (Fig. 6). With the obtained ϕ_{offset} from the former two correspondences, the algorithm can efficiently validate further point correspondences by comparing the angles between each already assigned point correspondence with the candidate point pair in both descriptors Q_R and Q_S. The assignment is rejected if a predefined angular difference λ_{th} is exceeded.

With regard to the example, the angles ϕ_{ac} and $\phi_{a'c'}$, and ϕ_{bc} and $\phi_{b'c'}$ are compared. If one of the differences $\phi_{diff_\alpha} = |(\phi_{a'c'} - \phi_{offset}) - \phi_{ac}|$ or $\phi_{diff_\beta} = |(\phi_{b'c'} - \phi_{offset}) - \phi_{bc}|$ is larger than the threshold λ_{th}, the assignment $c \leftrightarrow c'$ is rejected and the next correspondence pair $d \leftrightarrow c'$ is tested. Otherwise the algorithm tries to establish further point correspondences by following the same routine.

The PRM algorithm in this way can be formulated very compactly in a recursive manner. With every recursive step, one new point pair is tested and potentially rejected. The current best solution is the one which could determine most point correspondences. If several solutions have an equal number of correspondences, the one with the lowest accumulated angular difference is chosen.

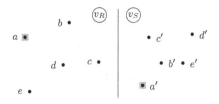

Fig. 4. The first correspondence assumption is marked in green. (Color figure online)

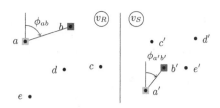

Fig. 5. The second correspondence assumption is marked in red. (Color figure online)

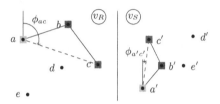

Fig. 6. The next correspondence is added and is marked in red. (Color figure online)

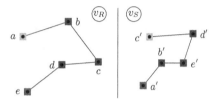

Fig. 7. Final solution to the correspondence problem.

With the angular threshold $\lambda_{th} \geq 360°$ and number of nearest neighbors N_{nb} = number of all points, the PRM algorithm corresponds to an exhaustive brute-force search of the best possible combination. The parameters λ_{th} and N_{nb} help pruning the exhaustive search tree significantly by removing branches with an unreasonably high error early in the recursive search and by limiting the search space. The final assigned solution for the given example can be seen in Fig. 7.

The bottom-up approach of PRM handles occluded points in a natural way. Since the algorithm tries to find corresponding point pairs locally, it will simply skip any occluded points and try to assign the next point in the list. The comparison of angles is facilitated with the use of the point set descriptors Q_R and Q_S as look-up tables. The only arithmetic computations during the recursion process are the subtraction of the angle offset ϕ_{offset} and accumulation of the angular error, the rest are just comparisons.

3   Experiments and Results

In all the experiments, the PRM uses an angular threshold $\lambda_{th} = 30°$ and considers $N_{nb} = 4$ neighbors.

PRM: Varying Camera Viewing Angle. In order to benchmark the PRM algorithm, we evaluated it on synthetic data in a *MATLAB* environment and compared it against a recently published method based on shape context and minimum spanning trees [7], denoted as SC.

The goal of this experiment was to assess the performance of the PPM algorithms with respect to the camera direction, thus varying projective distortion. The camera direction is always measured relative to the reference direction. For every sample camera direction, denoted as θ_{cap}, 5000 randomly selected camera positions within the range from $0°$ to θ_{cap} (Fig. 8) are generated and for each camera position a random point pattern consisting of nine 3D points is projected and tested. Whenever the sample θ_{cap} produces a correspondence match with at least 6 correct matches (minimum number of points required to compute the camera pose) with no mismatched points, the sample is considered as correct. The random point pattern is constrained to be in a rectangular volume of the same size as the points located on our real objects: 75 mm × 45 mm and 15 mm in depth relative to the reference direction.

The results are shown in Fig. 9. Between $0°$ and $5.5°$, SC shows better results. For larger viewing angles, PRM performs better.

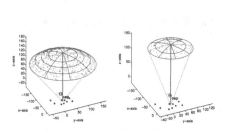

Fig. 8. Two different θ_{cap}. The reference direction is shown in blue, the red crosses on the spherical cap denote the random camera positions, and the blue dots represent a point pattern. (Color figure online)

Fig. 9. Success rate with varying camera viewing angle.

Computational Performance of the Android Implementation. The measurements were taken on an *Asus Transformer Prime TF 201, Tegra 3 1400 MHz*. The average times were determined using natural images as seen in the medical application described below. The mean time elapsed for reading an image from the camera required 10 ms whereas the segmentation on the GPU and CPU required 45 ms. Together with an average of 3 ms required for the PRM (C implementation) and some additional overhead to render the 3D object into the image, this resulted in an average framerate of 15 frames per second. A significant amount of time is required to pass data through the *Java Native Interface*.

Accuracy of the AR Navigation System. The accuracy was determined by measuring the distance between a real point and its augmented location. The measurement was performed in the image and converted to metric units. From six different camera positions, one measurement for each was done. A mean error of 0.8 mm between the real and the augmented position could be evaluated. The standard deviation was 1.0 mm with a maximum error of 2.6 mm.

4   Medical Application

Together with the surgeons, the applicability of the proposed technique was shown in-vitro for tumor surgeries in the head and neck area. The surgeon placed the markers in locations well identifiable in the MR/CT scan as well as on the anatomical models. Figures 10 and 11 show our Android navigation solution at execution with the tumor and other critical structures overlaid onto the image.

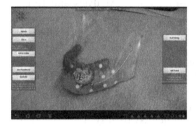
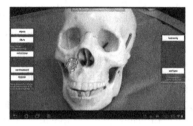

Fig. 10. A tumor in mandibulae region and the alveolaris nerve.

Fig. 11. A tumor in zygomaticum region and a missing tooth.

5   Discussion

The main conclusions that can be drawn from these experiments is that the PRM algorithm is more robust in comparison to the state-of-the-art in finding corresponding point pairs and is suitable for mobile real-time applications. Furthermore, the algorithm is based on a simple concept and can be implemented rather easily. The improved insensitivity, as compared to the state-of-the-art, to perspective changes, PRM lends itself to practical applications for example in clinical navigation tasks.

Although, the monte-carlo simulations showed a small disadvantage of PRM over SC for small perspective distortions, no such effect could be observed for real scenes.

A limitation common to all optical navigation solutions is the line of sight problem. During a surgical intervention landmarks can get covered for example by a surgical instrument or the hand of the surgeon. Once less than six landmarks can be seen no camera pose estimation is possible anymore. A further restriction is the rigid body assumption that is not valid in every case. Putting the landmarks on soft-tissue, for example skin, could thus pose additional challenges.

6   Conclusion

In this paper we proposed a single-view 3D navigation system applicable for general guidance tasks during surgeries. The achieved accuracy combined with its low cost opens a whole new field of easily deployable surgical navigation systems that could also find their application in third-world countries or in remote areas.

Beyond its clinical use, the introduced PPM algorithm performs well under perspective distortion and may contribute in general to AR applications on computational low-powered devices such as tablet computers or smartphones.

References

1. David, D., Duraiswami, S.: SoftPOSIT: simultaneous pose and correspondence determination. Int. J. Comput. Vision **59**(3), 259–284 (2004)
2. Denton, J., Beveridge, J.R.: Two dimensional projective point matching. In: Proceedings of the Fifth IEEE Southwest Symposium on Image Analysis and Interpretation 2002, pp. 77–81. IEEE (2002)
3. Goshtasby, A.A.: Point pattern matching. In: Image Registration, pp. 267–312 (2012)
4. Hofmann, R., Seichter, H., Reitmayr, G.: A gpgpu accelerated descriptor for mobile devices. In: 2012 IEEE International Symposium on Mixed and Augmented Reality (ISMAR), pp. 289–290. IEEE (2012)
5. Klein, G., Murray, D.: Parallel tracking and mapping on a camera phone. In: 8th IEEE International Symposium on Mixed and Augmented Reality, ISMAR 2009, pp. 83–86. IEEE (2009)
6. Kosmopoulos, V., Schizas, C.: Pedicle screw placement accuracy: a meta-analysis. Spine **32**(3), E111–E120 (2007)
7. Lian, W., Zhang, L., Zhang, D.: Rotation-invariant nonrigid point set matching in cluttered scenes. IEEE Trans. Image Process. **21**(5), 2786–2797 (2013)
8. McIlroy, P., Izadi, S., Fitzgibbon, A.: Kinectrack: agile 6-DoF tracking using a projected dot pattern. In: 2012 IEEE International Symposium on Mixed and Augmented Reality (ISMAR), pp. 23–29. IEEE (2012)
9. Oberst, M., Bertsch, C., Würstlin, S., Holz, U.: CT analysis of leg alignment after conventional vs. navigated knee prosthesis implantation. Initial results of a controlled, prospective and randomized study. Der Unfallchirurg **106**(11), 941 (2003)
10. Schweiger, F., Zeisl, B., Georgel, P., Schroth, G., Steinbach, E.,Navab, N.: Maximum detector response markers for SIFT and SURF. In: Int. Workshop on Vision, Modeling and Visualization (VMV), vol. 6 (2009)
11. Voss, K., Suesse, H.: Affine point pattern matching. In: Radig, B., Florczyk, S. (eds.) DAGM 2001. LNCS, vol. 2191, pp. 155–162. Springer, Heidelberg (2001)
12. WHO: Research for Patient Safety. http://www.who.int/patientsafety/information_centre/documents/ps_research_brochure_en.pdf (2008)

Structure-Guided Nonrigid Registration of CT–MR Pelvis Scans with Large Deformations in MR-Based Image Guided Radiation Therapy

David Rivest-Hénault[✉], Peter Greer, Jurgen Fripp, and Jason Dowling

CSIRO, Royal Brisbane and Women's Hospital, Herston, Queensland, Australia
david.rivest-henault@csiro.au

Abstract. Multimodal registration of CT and MR scans is a required step in leading edge adaptive MR-based image guided radiation therapy protocols. Yet, anatomical changes limit the precision of the registration process and therefore that of the whole intervention. In prostate radiation therapy, the difference in bladder and rectum filling can significantly displace both the targeted area and the organs at risk. Here, we describe a method that integrates an image-based similarity criterion with the anatomical information from manual contours to guide the registration process toward an accurate solution. Whole pelvis CT and MR scans of 33 patients have been nonrigidly registered, and the proposed method leads to an average improvement of 0.17 DSC when compared to a baseline nonrigid registrations. The increased accuracy will thus enhance an MR-based prostate radiation therapy protocol.

1 Introduction

The field of image guided radiation therapy (IMRT) is currently undergoing a strong push toward the establishment of MR-based clinical protocols. In prostate radiation therapy, in particular, the good soft tissue contrast of MRI brings clear clinical advantages: the prostate is much easier to identify and contour [11], which can result in reduced toxicity and improved treatment outcome. However, the problem of estimating the megavoltage attenuation coefficients from the MR images is a major hurdle preventing a widespread acceptance of MR-based protocols. This problem is also of the foremost importance in what concerns the assessment of toxicity following radiation therapy and in PET-MR imaging.

Currently, atlas-based methods are generally considered as the most accurate approaches [2] for the estimation of attenuation coefficient from MR. While atlas-based methods were first defined in the context of brain imaging [2], some authors recently reported promising result on pelvis imaging [5]. These methods rely on the availability of a multi-patient atlas composed of accurately registered CT and MR volumes in order to estimate an electron density mapping. However, CT–MRI co-registration of pelvis imaging remains a challenging task, even when

M. Erdt et al. (Eds.): CLIP 2013, LNCS 8361, pp. 65–73, 2014.
DOI: 10.1007/978-3-319-05666-1_9, © Springer International Publishing Switzerland 2014

considering only the simpler rigid and affine cases [4]. Moreover, the maximal accuracy achievable by atlas-based method is directly linked to the accuracy of the registration process in use. When rigid or affine registration is relied upon, any potentially large deformation of the anatomy — for example bladder filling or gas movement in the bowel — happening between the two imaging sessions will significantly limit the precision of the method. Hence, nonrigid registration is required to align CT and MR scans of the pelvis with high accuracy.

The large CT–MR image intensity discrepancy makes nonrigid registration challenging. For such multimodal problems, the mutual information (MI) criterion [10] is generally considered as the standard image similarity metric, but, in our experience, has too many local minima to drive the registration process to the optimal solution on its own. Several attempts to overcome this difficulty have been presented. For example, Andronache et al.[1] consider using a combination of both MI and CC and some intensity mapping function to solve various CT–MR registration problem, however they do not address directly the problem of large deformations. A semi-automatic method is considered by Fei et al. [6] which overcomes the challenge associated with large deformations by using a small number of fiducial points selected by an operator. Methods allowing a higher level of anatomical-prior integration were also proposed. The method recently presented by [8] uses the output of the automatic segmentation computed by FreeSurfer to guide a brain registration process. The method is designed to be very accurate for inter-subject registration, but its computational cost is currently prohibitive for our application, which is mostly focused on adaptive MR-based radiation therapy. In addition, no results on intermodal datasets are presented. In [7], the authors present a method for the registration of full body CT and MR scans that incorporates anatomical guidance by using prior knowledge on class probabilities. They use a Bayesian Approach to derive class probabilities from the MR intensity, and then use a Kullback-Leibler metric in the energy function to take this prior into account. However, they do not consider the integration prior information from previously defined automatic or manual contours.

This paper presents a new methodology that allows integrating the geometrical information provided by the different structure contours into the nonrigid registration process. Background information on nonrigid registration is provided in Sect. 2. Section 3 discusses the performance of classic nonrigid schemes and describes the proposed structure-guided nonrigid registration framework. The results of experiments conducted on a 33 patients CT–MR dataset are reported in Sect. 4. Finally, Sect. 5 holds a discussion and the conclusion.

2   Diffeomorphic CT–MR Nonrigid Registration

Nonrigid registration generally involves the optimization of some objective function composed of (1) an image similarity term, and (2) a regularization term. The former is a certain measure of how close the two images to be registered are, and the latter represents certain *a priori* concerning the form of the estimated deformation field. Formally, we have

$$E(I_1, I_2, \mathbf{T}) = E_{Sim}(I_1, \mathbf{T}(I_2)) - \lambda E_{Reg}(\mathbf{T}) \tag{1}$$

where $\mathbf{T}$ is a nonrigid transformation operation. Various transformation models were proposed in the literature each having different trade-off. The B-Spline based free-form transformation model presented by Rueckert et al. [13] was selected in this work since it is generally considered accurate, can be computed efficiently [9], and can be constrained to diffeomorphic mappings [14]. In CT–MR registration, there is no straightforward relation between the image intensities. The Mutual Information (MI) criterion and its normalized version (NMI) only assume that there is some sort of statistical relationship between the two images, and are now *de facto* standard in nonrigid multimodal registration. For an enlightening discussion of the subject, we refer the reader to [10]. In this work, we used $E_{Sim} = $ NMI. In what concerns regularization, we propose using the classic bending energy [13] term in conjunction with a term that ensures that the deformation field is diffeomorphic [9], as follows:

$$E_{Reg} = \frac{1}{V} \int_\Omega \|H(\mathbf{x})\|_F d\mathbf{x} + \epsilon \int_\Omega \log |J(\mathbf{x})| d\mathbf{x} \tag{2}$$

where V denotes the volume of the image domain Ω, $\mathbf{x} = (x, y, z)$, $|J(\mathbf{x})|$ is the determinant of the Jacobian matrix, and $\|H(\mathbf{x})\|_F$ is the Frobenius norm of the Hessian matrix. The first part favours smooth deformations. The second part penalizes the log of the Jacobian of the transformation. A Jacobian $|J|$ greater than 1 indicates an area of expansion in the deformation field, $|J| < 1$ indicates contraction, and $|J| <= 0$ indicates lost of information or folding and is a pathological case. The term $\log |J|$ goes to infinity as $|J|$ goes to 0, and, in fact, ensures that the deformation field is diffeomorphic. The final registration transformation $\mathbf{T}$ is computed by maximizing (1) using a pyramid approach [13].

3   Methodology

The nonrigid registration method discussed above has been demonstrated suitable for a large range of problems and can also be applied to CT–MR pelvis

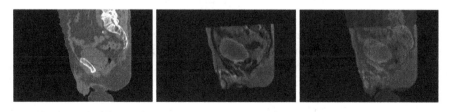

Fig. 1. Sample nonrigid registration using (1), sagittal planes. *From left to right*: CT scan, registered MR scan, and blended image. Note the difference in bladder size.

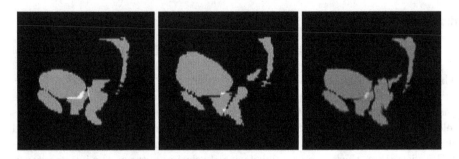

Fig. 2. Sample nonrigid contour registration for the following tissue: bladder, prostate, rectum, and bones using (3), sagittal planes. *From left to right*: reference CT contour, input MR contour, and MR contour after registration and resampling. Note how the registered MR bladder contours better matches that from the CT contours images.

registration with some success. However, as depicted in Fig. 1, the computed deformation is somewhat too local to allow to compensate for large deformation — in this case the change in bladder volume. This is a serious problem in prostate radiation therapy since the bladder volume can change significantly within a few minutes, thereby displacing the target (prostate) by several millimetres, and presumably reducing the efficiency of the treatment as well as augmenting toxicity.

3.1   Anatomical Prior

Tissue contours, either obtained as part of the standard clinical protocol, using an automatic method [3], or otherwise, can be used as strong geometric cues to guide the registration process. Given a collection of N pairs of CT–MR contours, a deformation field can be computed that maps the MR contours to the CT contours by optimizing the energy function

$$E(C_1, C_2, \mathbf{T}) = E_{Struc}(C_1, \mathbf{T}(C_2)) - \gamma E_{Reg}(\mathbf{T}) \qquad (3)$$

with

$$E_{Struc}(C_1, \mathbf{T}(C_2)) = \frac{1}{N} \sum_{i=1}^{N} \mathsf{S}(C_{1,i}, \mathbf{T}(C_{2,i})) \qquad (4)$$

where $\mathsf{S}(C_i, C_j)$ is some similarity measure. In this work, the contours are represented using binary volume where 0 indicates the background and 1 indicate the contoured tissues. Different similarity measures are suitable to register such binary image, but NMI appears to have good performance characteristics and was selected for its ease of implementation.

Following a successful optimization, the computed transformation $\mathbf{T}$ (Fig. 2) is a good approximation of the true deformation field, but cannot be expected to be highly accurate due to unavoidable variability in the contouring process or imaging characteristics. In particular, in prostate radiation therapy the CT will generally be contoured with the goal of radiation planning in mind. As such, some tissue classes might be voluntary oversegmented to account for some presumed microscopic spreads or simply in reason of the poor soft tissue contrast. The MR contours are generally closer to the true soft tissue anatomy, but bone contours are necessary inaccurate on T2 scans due to the very low signal. In addition, intra- or inter-rater variability will affect the results.

3.2 Structure-Guided Nonrigid Registration

Here, we propose an integrated method that allows for anatomical-guidance while taking into account the image intensity in the registration process. The main hypothesis in this method is that the contour can provide an initial solution, but that the maximization of the image similarity criterion will allow finding the best transformation. Using (1), (2), and (3), we define

$$E(I_1, I_2, C_1, C_2, \mathbf{T}) = (1 - \alpha)E_{Sim}(I_1, \mathbf{T}(I_2)) + \alpha E_{Struc}(C_1, \mathbf{T}(C_2))$$
$$- (\lambda(1 - \alpha) + \alpha\gamma)E_{Reg}(\mathbf{T}). \tag{5}$$

The parameter $\alpha \in [0, 1]$ adjusts the trade-off between anatomical guidance and the image similarity criterion, and might vary during the registration. Intuitively, we propose using α should be close to 1 at the beginning of the process, and reducing it to 0 at the final stage. Hence, at the end of the process, (5) reduces to (1), and the proposed method has not changed the optimization problem, but only the initial solution and search direction. As $\mathbf{T}$ as been selected to remain diffeomorphic throughout the registration process, no loss of information or unrealistic folding of the space occur at any step. It is worth noting that the factor $(\lambda(1 - \alpha) + \alpha\gamma)$ might be reduced to a constant, but this form is more explicit about the different numerical scales of E_{Sim} and E_{Struc}.

4 Experiments

A dataset of 33 CT–MR scans were acquired during the course of a study involving prostate cancer patients that have been prescribed hypofractionated radiation therapy. The CT scans were acquired with either a GE LightSpeed scanner with 2.0 mm slices or a Toshiba Acquilion scanner with 2.5 mm slices. MRIs were FSE-x1 T2 scans with a field of view encompassing the whole pelvis with 3.0 mm slices. A group of radiation oncologists and experience radiation therapists contoured the prostate, bladder, rectum and bones on all CT and MR scans. Before applying the presented nonrigid registration method, each MR scan has been preprocessed with the N3 algorithm [15] and aligned with the corresponding CT scan using a robust inverse-consistent affine registration algorithm [12].

Same-patient CT and MR scans were registered using the proposed structure-guided registration method corresponding to (5), and also with the NiftyReg [9] registration tool (adjusted according to (1)) for comparison purpose. The parameters of the method permit to adjust the smoothness of the registration transformation. Selecting the best parameters is non-trivial and problem dependant. Here, we selected the following set of parameters by trial and error: $\epsilon = 0.2, \lambda = 0.01, \gamma = 0.00125$. The last parameter, α balance the weight of the contour term. In this study, we decided to perform a two step optimization, first with $\alpha = 1$, and then with $\alpha = 0$. Hence, the final solution depends only on the image-based term. Evaluating the results is difficult as no ground-truth exist for this kind of problem. Still, we consider here three types of performance indicator: (1) qualitative result images, (2) the residual NMI, and (3) the Dice Similarity Criterion (DSC), as computed using the CT and MR manual contours. The last method is attractive since it relies on expert knowledge of the anatomy. However, it must be stressed that although the contours are not used at the last stage of the registration, they are still used at an earlier stage to provide structure-guidance. Therefore, this measure is biased toward the proposed method, and must be interpreted carefully. Nonetheless, we present it here since the position of those very structures is critical in radiation therapy. Sample result images are presented in Fig. 3, and quantitative results are in Table 1. Computational time for the structure-guided method was about 15 min per scan, which is reasonable for off-line CT-MR atlas construction.

5   Discussion and conclusion

The results presented in Table 1 and in Fig. 3 indicate that the proposed method leads to substantial improvements in the nonrigid registration of CT-MR images with potentially large deformations. However, as presented in Table 1, our method does not lead to a large improvement in the NMI between the CT and MR image. This constitutes an interesting manifestation of the multimodal nature of the NMI optimization surface: although the final registration transformation computed by the two methods might differ vastly, they both achieve a similar level in term of the similarity metric. Thus, the proposed method allows finding potentially more accurate local minima than the more traditional method. In the future, different values for alpha will also be explored, to see if the accuracy of the method can be improved. In addition, using multiple contours created by different observers will enable us to perform a fairer evaluation of the algorithms.

Table 1. Quantitative comparison of registration methods. Average values, 33 patients.

	Tissue	Affine [12]	NiftyReg [9]	Proposed
Dice	Bladder	0.6606	0.6559	0.8883
	Prostate	0.6196	0.6249	0.8212
	Rectum	0.5776	0.6020	0.8090
	Bones	0.7539	0.7682	0.8800
	Average	0.6529	0.6627	0.8496
	NMI	1.8977	1.8998	1.9015

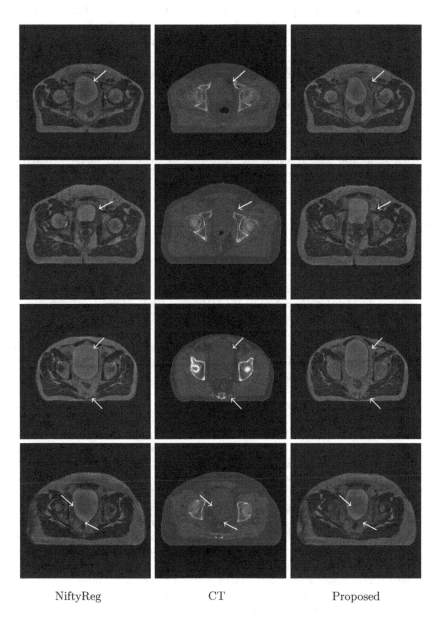

NiftyReg	CT	Proposed

Fig. 3. Sample results, axial view. Each row corresponds to a different patient. Note the improvements in bladder and rectum size and position (arrows). The MR images were resampled in the CT images space. *From left to right*: results obtained with NiftyReg, reference CT images, and results obtained with the proposed method.

To summarize, in this paper, we have presented a new methodology that allows integrating the geometrical information provided by different structure contours into the nonrigid registration process. The nonrigid transformation mapping an MR image to a CT image is estimated by optimizing an energy function that takes into account both image-based and contour-based similarity measures. Future work will include the integration of this structure-guided nonrigid registration scheme into an atlas-based method for electron density estimation from MR images.

Acknowledgments. This research was supported by the Cancer Council NSW (RG 11-05), the Prostate Cancer Foundation of Australia (YI2011), Movember and Cure Cancer Australia.

References

1. Andronache, A., von Siebenthal, M., Székely, G., Cattin, P.: Non-rigid registration of multi-modal images using both mutual information and cross-correlation. Med. Image Anal. **12**(1), 3–15 (2008)
2. Bezrukov, I., Mantlik, F., Schmidt, H.: MR-based PET attenuation correction for PET/MR imaging. Semin. Nucl. Med. **43**(1), 45–59 (2013)
3. Chandra, S.S., Dowling, J.A., Shen, K.K., Raniga, P., Pluim, J.P.W., Greer, P.B., Salvado, O., Fripp, J.: Patient Specific prostate segmentation in 3-D Magnetic Resonance Images. IEEE Trans. Med. Imag. **31**(10), 1955–1964 (2012)
4. Dean, C.J., Sykes, J.R., Cooper, R.A., Hatfield, P., Carey, B., Swift, S., Bacon, S.E., Thwaites, D., Sebag-Montefiore, D., Morgan, A.M.: An evaluation of four CT-MRI co-registration techniques for radiotherapy treatment planning of prone rectal cancer patients. Br. J. Radiol. **85**(1009), 61-8 (2012)
5. Dowling, J., Lambert, J., Parker, J., Salvado, O., Fripp, J., Capp, A., Wratten, C., Denham, J.W., Greer, P.B.: An atlas-based electron density mapping method for magnetic resonance imaging MRI-alone treatment planning and adaptive MRI-based prostate radiation therapy. Int. J. Radiat. Oncol. Biol. Physics **83**(1), e5–e11 (2012)
6. Fei, B., Duerk, J.L., Sodee, D.B., Wilson, D.L.: Semiautomatic nonrigid registration for the prostate and pelvic MR volumes. Acad. radiol. **12**(7), 815–824 (2005)
7. Hofmann, M., Schölkopf, B., Bezrukov, I., Cahill, N.: Incorporating prior knowledge on class probabilities into local similarity measures for intermodality image registration. In: Proceedings of the MICCAI 2009 Workshop on Probabilistic Models for Medical Image Analysis (PMMIA 2009), pp. 220–231 (2009)
8. Khan, A.R., Wang, L., Beg, M.F.: Multistructure large deformation diffeomorphic brain registration. IEEE TBME **60**(2), 544–553 (2013)
9. Modat, M., Ridgway, G.R., Taylor, Z.A., Lehmann, M., Barnes, J., Hawkes, D.J., Fox, N.C., Ourselin, S.: Fast free-form deformation using graphics processing units. Comput. Methods Programs Biomed. **98**(3), 278–284 (2010)
10. Pluim, J.P.W., Maintz, J.B.A., Viergever, M.A.: Mutual-information-based registration of medical images: a survey. IEEE TMI **22**(8), 986–1004 (2003)
11. Rasch, C., Barillot, I., Remeijer, P., Touw, A., van Herk, M., Lebesque, J.V.: Definition of the prostate in CT and MRI: a multi-observer study. Int. J. Radiat. Oncol. Biol. Physics **43**(1), 57–66 (1999)

12. Rivest-Henault, D., Dowson, N., Greer, P., Dowling, J.: Inverse-consistent rigid registration of CT and MR for MR-based planning and adaptive prostate radiation therapy. IOP Journal of Physics (2013) (accepted)
13. Rueckert, D., Sonoda, L.I., Hayes, C., Hill, D.L., Leach, M.O., Hawkes, D.J.: Non-rigid registration using free-form deformations: application to breast MR images. IEEE Trans. Med. Imag. **18**(8), 712–721 (1999)
14. Rueckert, D., Aljabar, P., Heckemann, R.A., Hajnal, J.V., Hammers, A.: Diffeo-morphic registration using B-splines. In: Larsen, R., Nielsen, M., Sporring, J. (eds.) MICCAI 2006. LNCS, vol. 4191, pp. 702–709. Springer, Heidelberg (2006)
15. Sled, J.G., Zijdenbos, A.P., Evans, A.C.: A nonparametric method for automatic correction of intensity nonuniformity in MRI data. IEEE Trans. Med. Imag. **17**(1), 87–97 (1998)

Placement of External Ventricular Drains Using an Average Model

I. Reinertsen[1,4](✉), A.S. Jakola[2,3,4], O. Solheim[2,3,4], F. Lindseth[1,2,4],
T. Selbekk[1,4], and G. Unsgaard[2,3,4]

[1] Department of Medical Technology, SINTEF, Trondheim, Norway
`Ingerid.Reinertsen@sintef.no`
[2] Norwegian University of Science and Technology (NTNU), Trondheim, Norway
[3] Department of Neurosurgery, St. Olav University Hospital, Trondheim, Norway
[4] National Competence Centre for Ultrasound and Image guided Therapy,
St. Olav University Hospital, Trondheim, Norway

Abstract. Purpose: Freehand placement of external ventricular drainage is not sufficiently accurate and precise. In the absence of high quality pre-operative 3D images, we propose the use of an average model for guidance of ventricular catheters. **Methods:** The model was segmented to extract the ventricles and registered to five normal volunteers. The proposed method was validated by comparing the trajectory resulting from the use of the average model to the use of volunteer-specific images. **Results:** The distances between the target points in the model and the volunteer-specific images at the left and right foramen of Monroe were computed (Mean±std: 5.74±1.39 mm and 6.00±1.17 mm for the left and right side respectively). We also compared the angles between the trajectories resulting from the use of volunteer specific data and the average model and the engagement of the trajectories with the frontal horn of the ipsilateral ventricle. **Conclusions:** Although an average model for guidance of a surgical procedure has a number of limitations, our initial experiments show that the use of a model might provide sufficient guidance for determination of the angle of insertion. Future work will include further clinical testing and possible refinement of the model.

Keywords: Image guided surgery · Neurosurgery · External ventricular drains

1 Introduction

Insertion of an external ventricular drain (EVD) is one of the most common procedures in neurosurgery. A small plastic catheter is placed inside the frontal horn of the lateral ventricle in order to relieve increased intracranial pressure or as part of a cerebral shunt in the treatment of hydrocephalus. The placement of an EDV is regarded as a fast and uncomplicated procedure often performed under emergency conditions either in the operating room or in the intensive care

M. Erdt et al. (Eds.): CLIP 2013, LNCS 8361, pp. 74–82, 2014.
DOI: 10.1007/978-3-319-05666-1_10, © Springer International Publishing Switzerland 2014

unit without rigid head fixation or three-dimensional pre-operative images. In general, only a few 2D CT images of the patient are available before surgery. The standard surgical technique is a freehand pass through a burr hole in the skull. The point of entry, called Kocher's point, is located approximately 1.5 cm anterior to the coronal suture and 2.5 cm lateral to the midline. The choice of trajectory to reach the frontal horn of the lateral ventricle is based on external landmarks such as the canthus of the eye and the tragus. Free flow of cerebrospinal fluid (CSF) from the distal end of the catheter is considered an indication of satisfactory placement. Unfortunately, occlusion of the catheter due to incorrect or sub-optimal placement is a major cause of re-operations and complications related to the procedure. Toma et al. [1] reported that only about 40 % of the 183 ventricular catheters in their retrospective study were correctly placed within the frontal horn of the lateral ventricle. Huyette et al. [2] retrospectively evaluated post-operative CT scans from 97 patients and found that only 56.1 % of the catheters were placed in the ipsi-lateral ventricle. They also found that 22.4 % of the catheters were placed in non-ventricular spaces. Even the successfully placed catheters were on average 16 mm from the target just above the foramen of Monroe. On average, two passes were needed for successful placement.

As the fraction of catheters incorrectly or sub-optimally placed remains high, different image guidance techniques have been developed. Hayhust et al. [3] developed and evaluated a system based on an electromagnetic positioning system. They concluded that image guidance reduced poor placement of the catheter and resulted in a significant decrease in the early shunt revision rate. Levitt et al. [4] also found that the accuracy of catheter placement was significantly improved with image guidance in a retrospective study of 102 shunt surgeries in 89 patients.

Even though image guidance seems to improve the accuracy of the catheter placement, the need for additional imaging and rigid head fixation makes the solution unattractive or even unfeasible in many cases, as pointed out by Kestle [5]. In this paper, we therefore investigate the use of a pre-defined model to guide the placement of ventricular catheters in the absence of patient-specific 3D images suited for traditional image guidance. The model is an adapted version of the ICBM152 non-linear symmetric average model [6]. Atlases and average models have traditionally been used in neurosurgery to guide procedures such as electrode placement for deep brain stimulation [7,8]. The atlas is then registered to a patient specific image in order to identify regions that are unresolved by conventional MRI imaging such as the nuclei of the basal ganglia and thalamus. In this paper, however, we use the average model directly to guide the placement of ventricular catheters. The model is registered to the patient using a set of anatomical landmarks in addition to a surface trajectory acquired with a computer tracked pointer on the patient's head. The registered model can then be used to plan the trajectory toward the ipsi-lateral ventricle and the foramen of Monroe. We have validated this approach using data from five normal volunteers, and we compare two trajectories starting from Kocher's point: (I) image guidance using volunteer specific data and (II) image guidance using model data, which is the new method proposed in this paper. The new model-based method and the validation experiments are detailed in the following sections.

2 Methods

2.1 Model Segmentation and Image-to-Volunteer Registration

The ICBM-152 average brain model was segmented using the Freesurfer package, which is documented and freely available for download online (http://surfer.nmr. mgh.harvard.edu/). The automatic segmentation of brain structures is described in Fischl et al. [9]. Following the full brain segmentation, we extracted the labels corresponding to the left and right lateral ventricles and the third ventricle. The third ventricle is important in order to clearly see the foramen of Monroe which is the target point for the placement of ventricular catheters. We then segmented the skin surface from the model using the foreground filter that is part of 3DSlicer [10] (http://www.slicer.org/). This method uses the Otsu threshold algorithm [11] and morphological operators to achieve segmentation.

For validation purposes, we obtained T1-weighted MR images of the five normal volunteers that participated in the study. The MR images of the volunteers were also segmented using the Freesurfer package. The ventricles were extracted from the label dataset and the skin surfaces were segmented using the foreground filter in 3DSlicer. We also manually identified seven anatomical landmarks (lateral and medial canthus of both eyes, the nasion and tragus on each side) in each volunteers image volume.

2.2 Identification of Skin Landmarks in the Average Model

The use of anatomical landmarks for model-to-patient registration requires identification of anatomical skin landmarks in the ICBM-152 average brain. When the ICBM-152 average brain was generated [6], the optimization of the registration parameters was performed only on the brain. The skin, skull, eyes, muscles etc. were excluded from the registration algorithm using a brain mask. Consequently, the skin surface in the ICBM-152 average brain is blurry and reliable identification of anatomical skin landmarks in this volume is associated with considerable uncertainty. We therefore identified the seven anatomical landmarks in the MR images of the five volunteers. The MR images of the volunteers were then registered to the ICBM-152 average brain using the elastix software [12] built on top the InsightToolkit (ITK) [13]. In a first step, we performed a rigid body registration and then in a second step a full 12 parameters affine registration. In both steps we used the mutual information similarity measure and a standard gradient descent optimization technique. In general, non-linear registration is needed to accurately register an individual brain to the ICBM-152 average. In this case, we were mainly interested in registration of non-brain features such as the eyes and ears. We therefore considered an affine transformation to be sufficient for this purpose. The resulting transforms were then applied to the anatomical landmarks identified for the five volunteers bringing the landmarks into the ICBM-152 space. The landmarks corresponding to each anatomical location from the five volunteers were then averaged to generate seven landmarks in ICBM-152 space. The fact that the skin surface in the ICBM-152 average brain is blurry obviously represents a source of uncertainty in the segmentation of the skin surface. Therefore, we optimized the parameters of the skin surface segmentation in order to minimize the distance between the segmented surface and the anatomical landmarks. The mean distance between the points and the surface is 1.14 ± 0.53 mm.

2.3   Registration and Identification of Entry Point

Following skin surface segmentation and identification of anatomical landmarks, registration of the ICBM-152 average brain to the volunteer could be performed. In a first step, we used a tracked pointer (Northern Digital Inc., Waterloo, ON) to identify the seven anatomical points on the volunteer. We then continuously sampled points with the tracked pointer by moving the pointer tip over the available skin surface (face and scalp). For surface based registration, we use a modified version of the ICP [14] algorithm incorporating the least trimmed squares (LTS) estimator [15] to reduce the influence of possible outliers. More details can be found in [16]. In order to improve the accuracy we measured the maximum distance between the frontal horns of the ventricles in the volunteer-specific data and applied the corresponding scaling factor to the ventricles segmented from the model. This measurement is routinely performed by the neurosurgeons before the procedure in order to characterize the size of the ventricular system.

The standard entry point for EDV, called Kocher's point is located approximately 1.5 cm anterior to the coronal suture and 2.5 cm lateral to the midline. Definitions of this point may vary slightly, but we believe this definition is widely used among neurosurgeons. In order to construct the catheter trajectories we needed to locate this point in the volunteer datasets. Unfortunately, the coronal suture is not easily detected in T1-weighted MR images. Therefore, we used a result from Sarmento et al. [17] who investigated the relationship between the central lobe and the coronal suture in 32 cadavers. They found that the coronal suture was, on average, located 5.91 cm anterior to the central sulcus in the midline. We thus identified Kocher's point 5.91 cm + 1.5 cm = 7.41 cm anterior to the top of the central sulcus and 2.5 cm lateral to the midline on the right side in standard stereotactic space using the ICBM-152 average brain. As part of the segmentation using Freesurfer, the five datasets were registered to stereotactic space. It was therefore straightforward to invert these transforms in order to obtain Kocher's point in the native space of each dataset. Finally, the five Kocher's points were transformed using the image-to-volunteer registration in order to bring the entry points into the coordinate system of each volunteer.

2.4   Trajectories

In this paper, we compare two different trajectories starting at Kocher's point: (I) This is the trajectory from Kocher's point to the target defined at the foramen of Monroe in the volunteer-specific data registered to he volunteer. This trajectory does not represent the absolute truth as we do not take into account the registration error between the image and the volunteer. Consequently, this trajectory represents the use of traditional neuronavigation for placement of ventricular catheters. (II) Second, the model-based trajectory is the trajectory from Kocher's point to the target defined at the foramen of Monroe in the average model registered to the volunteer. This is the new trajectory we propose in this paper.

3   Experiments

We validated the method on five normal volunteers. The volunteers were placed in a supine position. The head was immobilized using a vacuum pillow routinely used for shunt patients. Using our in-house navigation system with an optical tracking system (Polaris, Northern Digital Inc., Waterloo, ON), we acquired the position of the seven anatomical landmarks using a tracked pointer: lateral and medial canthus of both eyes, the nasion and tragus on each side. We finally acquired a set of surface points by continuously sampling a trajectory on the skin surface.

Using the image-to-patient registration method described in Sect. 2.3, we retrospectively registered the ICBM-152 average brain to the volunteer. We used a seven parameters linear transformation (3 translations, 3 rotations and isotropic scaling). The landmarks corresponding to the volunteer in question were excluded from the average point set in model space in order to avoid any bias. The resulting transformation was also applied to the segmented ventricles. In order to validate the position and orientation of the resulting ventricles, we used the T1-weighted MR image of the volunteer. We registered the volunteer-specific dataset to the volunteer in a similar manner. For this registration, we used a rigid body transformation. The resulting transformation was finally applied to the segmented volunteer-specific ventricles. Following image-to-volunteer registration we determined the position of Kocher's point in each dataset and constructed the two trajectories starting at this point for each volunteer. We also identified the target points for a ventricular catheter in each lateral ventricle immediately above the foramen of Monroe and computed the distances between the target points in the average model and the volunteer-specific datasets.

4   Results

To evaluate the accuracy of the average model we measured the distance between the target points in the average model and in the volunteer-specific dataset. The results are presented in Table 1. In order to compare the two trajectories,

Table 1. Distances between the target points (left and right foramen of Monroe) in the average model and the volunteer-specific datasets

Volunteer	Distance left targets (mm)	Distance right targets(mm)
1	4.67	5.23
2	7.06	6.71
3	6.13	6.67
4	3.91	4.32
5	6.92	7.08
Mean±std (mm)	5.74±1.39	6.00±1.17

Table 2. Angles between volunteer specific and model based trajectories for five volunteers.

Volunteer	Angle (degree)
1	3.77
2	4.47
3	4.00
4	2.14
5	3.53
Mean±std	3.58±0.88

Table 3. The length of the different trajectories (mm) inside the frontal horn of the right lateral ventricle

Volunteer	Volunteer specific	Model
1	14.65	10.63
2	13.40	10.90
3	25.00	23.15
4	16.80	14.66
5	19.90	15.50
Mean±std	17.9±4.64	14.97±5.07

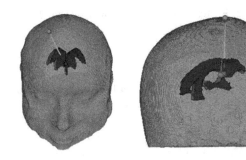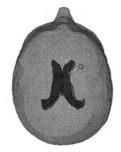

Fig. 1. The different trajectories constructed for one of the volunteers: Volunteer-specific ventricles in orange, model ventricles in blue, Kocher's point in green, volunteer specific trajectory in green and model based trajectory in yellow (Color figure online).

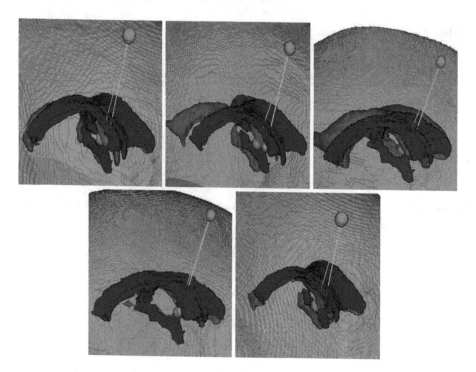

Fig. 2. The different trajectories for all five volunteers: Volunteer-specific ventricles in orange, model ventricles in blue, Kocher's point in green, volunteer specific trajectory in green and model-based trajectory in yellow (Color figure online).

we computed the angle between the volunteer specific trajectory and the model-based trajectory. The results are given in Table 2. We also computed the length of each trajectory inside the frontal horn of the volunteer-specific right lateral ventricle in mm. These results are presented in Table 3. The model-based trajectory intersects with the frontal horn of the lateral ventricle in all five cases. An example of the two trajectories in one volunteer is shown in Fig. 1 and a closer view of the trajectories and ventricles in all five datasets is shown in Fig. 2.

5   Discussion and Conclusions

In this paper, we have presented the use of an average model to guide the placement of ventricular catheters in the brain. We have validated the method using data from five normal volunteers and compared guidance using the ICBM-152 average brain to the use of volunteer specific data. In this limited and preliminary study, we have shown that it is possible to obtain a registration error on the order of 6 mm at the foramen of Monroe and a deviation in the angle compared to the use of patient specific data below 4°. These results suggest that the average model could provide sufficiently accurate guidance for this procedure. In the placement of EVDs a placement is often considered successful if the tip of the catheter is free-floating inside the frontal horn of the ventricle. The engagement of the trajectory with the ventricle is therefore important to ensure a free-floating catheter tip. The results presented here show that the engagement of the model based trajectory will ensure an engagement similar to the trajectory based on volunteer specific data. Volunteer-specific data in this context do not represent the absolute truth, but rather the use of a conventional neuro-navigation system with associated registration errors.

Compared to the freehand method, almost any means of guidance will improve the accuracy and precision of the procedure. The challenge will be to keep the solution simple and fast in order to avoid the introduction of perceived obstacles in an otherwise quick and simple procedure. Obviously, the use of an average model present a number of limitations, but in the absence of 3D pre-operative images, this study suggest that a model might be sufficiently accurate for planning the entry point and the trajectory of the catheter. Further development of the model and more extensive validation are required in order to evaluate the accuracy and precision of the method when applied to clinical datasets. Most EVDs are performed on patients with enlarged ventricles. Normal sized ventricles therefore represent relatively challenging cases in this context. Still, the accuracy of the model could be further improved by incorporating other patient-specific parameters routinely used such as midline shift. An additional possibility is to combine the use of an average model with intra-operative ultrasound as suggested in [18] in order to have even more patient specific information about the size, shape, position and orientation of the ventricles.

References

1. Toma, A.K., et al.: External ventricular drain insertion accuracy: is there a need for change in practice? Neurosurgery **65**(6), 1197–1201 (2009)
2. Huyette, D.R., et al.: Accuracy of the freehand pass technique for ventriculostomy catheter placement: retrospective assessment using computer tomography scans. J. Neurosurg. **108**, 88–91 (2008)
3. Hayhurst, C., et al.: Effect of electromagnetic-navigated shunt placement on failure rates: a prospective multicenter study. J. Neurosurg. **113**, 1273–1278 (2010)
4. Levitt, M.R., et al.: Image-guided cerebrospinal fluid shunting in children: catheter accuracy and shunt survival. J. Neurosurg. Pediatr. **10**, 112–117 (2012)
5. Kestle, R.W.: Editorial: shunt malfunction. J. Neurosurg. **113**, 1270–1272 (2010)
6. Fonov, V.S., et al.: Unbiased average age-appropriate atlases for pediatric studies. NeuroImage **54**(1), 313–327 (2011)
7. Sadikot, A.F., et al.: Creation of computerized 3D MRI-integrated atlases of the human basal ganglia and thalamus. Front. Syst. Neurosci. **5**, 71 (2011)
8. Krauth, A., et al.: A mean three-dimensional atlas of the human thalamus: generation from multiple histological data. Front. Syst. Neurosci. **49**(3), 2053–2062 (2010)
9. Fischl, B., et al.: Sequence-independent segmentation of magnetic resonance images. NeuroImage **23**(Suppl. 1), S69–S84 (2004a)

10. Pieper, S., et al.: The NA-MIC kit: ITK, VTK, pipelines, grids and 3D slicer as an open platform for the medical image computing community. Proc. IEEE Int. Symp. Biomed. Imaging: From Nano to Macro **1**, 698–701 (2006)
11. Otsu, N.: A threshold selection method from gray-level histograms. IEEE Trans. Syst. Man Cybern. **9**(1), 62–66 (1979)
12. Klein, S., et al.: Elastix: a toolbox for intensity-based medical image registration. IEEE Trans. Med. Imaging. **29**, 196–205 (2010)
13. Ibanez, L., et al.: The ITK Software Guide: The Insight Segmentation and Registration Toolkit. Kitware Inc., New York (2005)
14. Besl, P.J., et al.: A method for registration of 3D shapes. IEEE Trans. Pattern Anal. Mach. Intell. **14**, 239–256 (1992)
15. Rousseeuw, P.J., et al.: Robust Regression and Outlier Detection. Wiley, New York (1987)
16. Reinertsen, I., Jakola, A., Solheim, O., Lindseth, F., Unsgård, G.: Model-guided placement of cerebral ventricular catheters. In: Barratt, D., Cotin, S., Fichtinger, G., Jannin, P., Navab, N. (eds.) IPCAI 2013. LNCS, vol. 7915, pp. 30–39. Springer, Heidelberg (2013)
17. Sarmento, S.A., et al.: Relationship between the coronal suture and the central lobe. Arq. Neuropsiquiatr. **66**(4), 868–871 (2008)
18. Reinertsen, I., et al.: A new system for 3D ultrasound-guided placement of cerebral ventricle catheters. IJCARS **7**(1), 151–157 (2012)

Automated Kidney Detection and Segmentation in 3D Ultrasound

Matthias Noll[✉], Xin Li, and Stefan Wesarg

Cognitive Computing and Medical Imaging, Fraunhofer IGD,
Fraunhoferstr. 5, Darmstadt, Germany
{matthias.noll,li.xin,stefan.wesarg}@igd.fraunhofer.de
http://www.igd.fraunhofer.de/en/Institut/Abteilungen/
Cognitive-Computing-Medical-Imaging

Abstract. Ultrasound provides the physical capabilities for a fast and save disease diagnosis in various medical scenarios including renal exams and patient trauma assessment. However, the experience of the ultrasound operator is the key element in performing ultrasound diagnosis. Thus, we like to introduce our automatic kidney detection and segmentation algorithm for 3D ultrasound. The approach utilizes basic kidney shape information to detect the kidney position. Following, the Level Set algorithm is applied to segment the detection result. In combination this method may help physicians and inexperienced trainees to achieve kidney detection and segmentation for diagnostic purposes.

Keywords: Ultrasound · Image analysis · Kidney · Shape prior · Detection · Segmentation

1 Introduction

Ultrasound is a widespread medical imaging system that provides a fast, non-invasive and non-hazardous way to obtain patient anatomy information. Despite its importance in medicine there are some challenges that have to be addressed when dealing with ultrasound images. Speckle, artifacts and generally a poor signal-to-noise ratio highly influence the image quality [7] and are therefore the hardest challenges to overcome. Additionally, the specific ultrasound intensity values fluctuate between consecutive recordings and vary even strongly between miscellaneous ultrasound devices. Thus, physicians or medical technicians are given multiple ways to manipulate the imaging output to their individual preferences. All these factors have to be addressed when designing automatic ultrasound image analysis algorithms.

Currently, most ultrasound diagnosis are still performed using 2D ultrasound technology. This is because physicians are accustomed to the standard ultrasound modality. If 3D ultrasound is available, it is often only used to acquire patient recordings for later review. All 3D datasets including CT and MRI are commonly presented using cross section views with sliced volume information,

M. Erdt et al. (Eds.): CLIP 2013, LNCS 8361, pp. 83–90, 2014.
DOI: 10.1007/978-3-319-05666-1_11, © Springer International Publishing Switzerland 2014

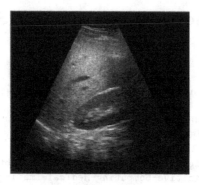

Fig. 1. eFAST recording of the right kindey. The image also includes the liver, the hepatorenal recess and a rib shadow extension (right).

which is hard to apply and work with in a live imaging systems like ultrasound [1]. A computer algorithm however can work directly on the 3D data.

The goal of this study was to design an automated kidney detection and segmentation method that utilizes the more and more available 3D ultrasound capability of ultrasound devices. The kidney is the target structure in this study, because it is frequently examined using ultrasound. Also, it has a unique bean-shape structure that is reasonably well recognizable by the human eye.

The kidneys are retroperitoneal organs that are protected by the lower ribs. Depending which kidney is the examination target, a recording is performed by placing the ultrasound transducer between the 5th to 9th intercostal space. During the exam the ultrasonographer must adhere the ribs, because they cause large shadow artifacts in the ultrasound that cannot be compensated during image processing. The right kidney is located just below the liver (see Fig. 1). Similar, the left kidney lies just below the spleen. Each kidney has a tough fibrous outer cortex that appears dark in the ultrasound. The inner renal sinus containing the renal pelvis with larger blood vessels, lymphatics and fatty tissue generates a brighter ultrasound echo, giving a good contrast to the outer cortex. Detecting and segmenting the kidney in ultrasound images could help in automating medical examination protocols like renal exams and eFAST. Also, this could help in creating an automated abdominal ultrasound diagnostic system.

2   Image Processing

2.1   Data Preparation and Pre-processing

Addressing the challenges mentioned in the introduction and generally enhance algorithm reproducibility, the influence of the image quality to the detection and segmentation is reduced [3]. We apply a multi-scale image pyramid (Fig. 2(a)) to the ultrasound, thereby reducing speckle and smoothing the image while preserving important larger abdominal structures [10]. Additionally, we adjust the

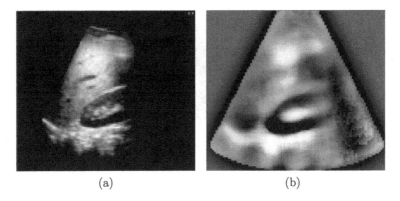

(a)   (b)

Fig. 2. (a) Downscaling of the input image. (b) Histogram equalized image with distinctive kidney shape

global image contrast through histogram equalization [8] (cf. Fig. 2(b)). This step is very time consuming and should be replaced with a more efficient alternative. We apply histogram equalization to decrease the image intensity fluctuations between different ultrasound recordings. For a kidney recording, the equalization result will usually contain the distinctive kidney shape composed of low intensity values.

After pre-processing we assume a bi-modal histogram composition for the equalization result. Applying Otsu's method to the equalized image calculates the optimum image threshold by minimizing the intra-class variance, thereby automatically reducing the gray level intensity image to a binary representation [6]. As a result, we obtain a "kidney candidate image" (Fig. 3), containing all possible kidney locations. The dark kidneys outer cortex is represented with a binary *one*, while the inner sinus receives a binary *zero* value.

We generalize the algorithm further, by applying additional information about the segmentation target e.g. the kidney shape. Here, we chose a 3D ellipsoid structure element, that represents a rough shape approximation of the kidneys inner sinus (Fig. 4). The structure element size is $20 \times 10 \times 10$ mm, so it

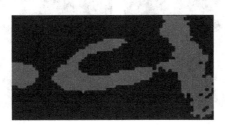

Fig. 3. Kidney candidate image showing the kidney location with the kidneys outer cortex (red) and inner sinus (black). Also visible on the right a recorded rib shadow creating a candidate artifact (Color figure online).

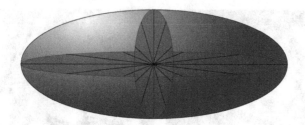

Fig. 4. Kidney structure element (shape prior). For simplicity the emitted rays (black) are illustrated for just two image directions.

will fit inside the kidney and especially inside the average renal pelvis. This is beneficial for the graph based search that is performed in the kidney detection step described in the next section. After the "structure element" selection we are able to utilize both signal and shape information during the image analysis. Advancing the algorithm in future implementations the simple structure element can be substituted by e.g. a model of the kidney sinus to gain specific shape information [9].

2.2 Detection

After the image pre-processing the kidney location is identified as follows. Initially, a search graph is constructed and applied to the kidney candidate image (Fig. 5(a)). The inter graph node step size is derived from the structure elements extent. The kidney structure element is then placed at each graph node. This way all possible kidney locations are investigated. In each step the structure element emits radial rays to each of the three image coordinate planes (see Fig. 5(b)). For a travel distance of 1.5× the structure elements diameter in emission direction and using m discrete detection steps, each emitted ray r_j ascertains the presence of zero-one crossings in the binary kidney candidate image. Here, we

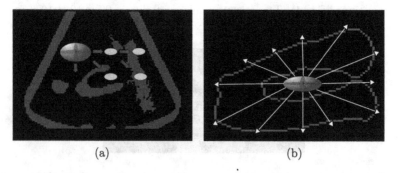

(a)   (b)

Fig. 5. (a) Graph-based searching using the kidney shape element on the kidney candidate image. (b) Detection of zero-crossings at the kidney position illustrated for the xy-image axis

utilize the differences in echogenicity between the inner and outer kidney fiber structures to detect the crossing from the renal pelvis to the outer cortex. Using the chosen structure element and the eFAST acquisition protocol, slight kidney rotations can be neglected. Strong rotations however will require an initial volume alignment. Each ray r_j with a detected zero-one crossing receives a ray score $f(i,j) = 1$, whereas the remaining rays receive a score of $f(i,j) = 0$. The kidney candidate with a score

$$S_c = \frac{\sum_{\substack{1<i\leq n \\ 1<j\leq n}} f(i,j)}{n}, \ f(i,j) \in [0,1] \tag{1}$$

of 80 % or more corresponds to the kidney position (cf. Fig. 6). A candidate score $S_c < 80$ % lead in some of the available test data to a false kidney detection at the ultrasound boundary. The score threshold parameter might be ultrasound device related and might need adjustment for other devices. Our tests showed further, that a number of $n = 12$ rays per image coordinate plane is sufficient to successfully detect the kidney location. Using more rays is always possible but ultimately will increases algorithm computation time. The candidate score would need adjustment. For recordings containing a rib shadow, using less than 12 rays lead to a false kidney detection. If more than one candidate achieves a score of 80 % or more, the candidate with the highest valid ray count is selected as the valid kidney position. Hence, the presented detection method will generate at most one kidney position. A successful graph search directly triggers the automated segmentation on the detection result.

2.3   Segmentation

For the remaining kidney candidate, each valid ray generates a seed point for the kidney segmentation. Here, the seed points are placed with an offset d to the detected crossing point along the rays direction. The offset d was chosen to be approximately haft the diameter of the kidneys outer cortex. Following, the fast marching algorithm [4] is applied to the collection of seed points to generate an intermediate kidney segmentation. The fast marching algorithm is a basic segmentation algorithm that uses a constant segmentation propagation speed and predefined iteration steps. It also requires a speed function to restrict the

Candidate   **Searching structure**   **Outlier removal**

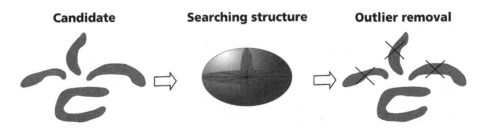

Fig. 6. Candidate search removes all invalid kidney candidates.

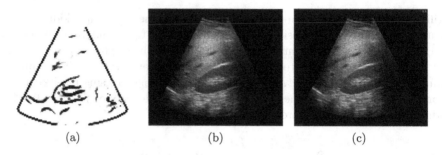

(a)   (b)   (c)

Fig. 7. Figure (a) shows the utilized speed function image (sigmoid) with indicated seed point placements. Figure (b) shows the intermediate segmentation result of the fast marching algorithm. The final segmentation result (b) was achieved by applying the Level Set algorithm.

segmentation propagation. We utilized a sigmoid computation of the histogram equalized input as the speed function (see Fig. 7(a)).

Because of this, the segmentation results are not always connected for all seed point areas (Fig. 7(b)). To achieve full segmentation connectivity we additionally apply the Level Set algorithm [2] to the intermediate fast marching segmentation result. The sigmoid image is once again used as the restricting speed function. The Level Set algorithm improved the segmentation result for most of the available test cases by connecting separated areas (cf. Fig. 7(c)). The output of the Level Set algorithm is the final segmentation result.

3   Results

We performed our experiments on 62 three-dimensional ultrasound data sets of 8 healthy male and female volunteers. The images were acquired using the right upper quadrant view of the eFAST exam. The kidney detection rate on the available data was above 90 %. The kidney could not be automatically detected in six data sets due to strong rib shadows, that cut through the kidney location. Here, no kidney candidate achieved the necessary 80 % valid rays criterion, because the shadow area included a large amount of image information about the inner kidney structure. The connection of kidney candidates to shadow artifacts (see Fig. 3) did not influence the detection result in the available test cases. However, avoiding rib shadows is still the most important task in acquiring data for the presented method. Due to this, we also implemented a shadow detection algorithm based on [5] to indicate the viability of an ultrasound recording for kidney detection.

The segmentation method was applied to the remaining 56 data sets, after the kidney detection generated a valid candidate. Some of the results are shown in (Fig. 8). However, the segmentation algorithm currently does not work properly in all of the available cases. In some images the Level Set leaked the kidney because of weak boundary gradients at the kidneys renal capsule. Here, the

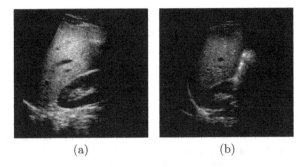

(a)   (b)

Fig. 8. Two example results of the proposed automated detection and segmentation method. In figure (b) a minor segmentation leak can be observed.

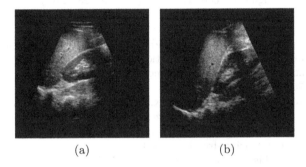

(a)   (b)

Fig. 9. Leaking Level Set results. Most commonly a leaking occurs at the threshold of a rib shadow (a). Figure (b) shows the worst leakage example of all 62 test data sets.

applied speed function did not generate the necessary restriction parameters to keep the algorithm from propagating the segmentation to the liver and other surrounding tissue. In (Fig. 9) we can see examples of the Level Set leaking the kidney with (Fig. 9(b)) being the worst result we achieved using the presented segmentation approach. Overall we are satisfied with the so far achieved results and we will continue working to improve the segmentation algorithm.

4   Conclusion

A method for automated kidney detection and segmentation in 3D ultrasound has been proposed. Both ultrasound image intensities and kidney shape priors in form of a structure element have been used in the process. The automated kidney detection was possible in all available data sets with no rib shadows. The kidney segmentation based on the detection results is feasible but has to be improved using more sophisticated algorithms before automatic diagnosis based on the segmentation result is achievable. We also believe, that the presence of a kidney can be excluded, if the number candidate score S_c does not exceed a certain threshold. We will investigate this possibility in further experiments with a greater variety of test data sets. We further need to investigate kidney pathologies because the assumption of finding the bright inner sinus versus the dark outer cortex might not hold.

References

1. Aliakseyeu, D., Subramanian, S., Martens, J.B., Rauterberg, M.: Interaction techniques for navigation through and manipulation of 2d and 3d data. In: Proceedings of the Workshop on Virtual Environments, EGVE '02, pp. 179–188. Eurographics Association, Aire-la-Ville, Switzerland, Switzerland (2002)
2. Chen, T.F.: Medical Image Segmentation Using Level Sets, pp. 1–8 (2008)
3. Contreras Ortiz, S.H., Chiu, T., Fox, M.D.: Ultrasound image enhancement: a review. Biomed. Signal Process. Control $7(5)$, 419–428 (2012)
4. Forcadel, N., Guyader, C., Gout, C.: Generalized fast marching method: applications to image segmentation $48(1$–$3)$, 189–211 (2008)
5. Hellier, P., Coupe, P., Meyer, P., Morandi, X., Collins, D.: Acoustic shadows detection, application to accurate reconstruction of 3d intraoperative ultrasound. In: 5th IEEE International Symposium on Biomedical Imaging: From Nano to Macro, ISBI 2008, pp. 1569–1572 (2008)
6. Hiransakolwong, N., Hua, K.A., Vu, K., Windyga, P.S.: Segmentation of ultrasound liver images: an automatic approach. In: Proceedings of the 2003 International Conference on Multimedia and Expo - ICME '03, vol. 2, pp. 573–576. IEEE Computer Society, Washington, DC (2003)
7. Loizou, C., Pattichis, C., Istepanian, R., Pantziaris, M., Kyriakou, E., Tyllis, T., Nicolaides, A.: Ultrasound image quality evaluation. In: 4th International IEEE EMBS Special Topic Conference on Information Technology Applications in Biomedicine, pp. 138–141 (2003)
8. Peng, B., Wang, Y., Yang, X.: A multiscale morphological approach to local contrast enhancement for ultrasound images. In: Proceedings of the 2010 International Conference on Computational and Information Sciences, ICCIS '10, pp. 1142–1145. IEEE Computer Society, Washington, DC (2010).
9. Xie, J., Jiang, Y., Tsui, H.T.: Segmentation of kidney from ultrasound images based on texture and shape priors. IEEE Trans. Med. Imag. $24(1)$, 45–57 (2005)
10. Zong, X., Laine, A.F., Geiser, E.A.: Speckle reduction and contrast enhancement of echocardiograms via multiscale nonlinear processing. IEEE Trans. Med. Imag. $17(4)$, 532–540 (1998)

Surgical Workflow Analysis, Design and Development of an Image-Based Navigation System for Endoscopic Interventions

Frederic Perez[1]([⊠]), Sergio Vera[1], Gloria Fernández-Esparrach[2],
Henry Córdova[2], Raúl San José Estépar[3], Javier Herrero Jover[1],
and Miguel Angel González Ballester[1]

[1] Alma IT Systems, Barcelona, Spain
frederic.perez@alma3d.com
[2] Endoscopy Unit, Department of Gastroenterology, Hospital Clinic,
Barcelona, Spain
[3] Harvard Medical School, Boston, MA, USA

Abstract. Endoscopic interventions in the abdominal and thoracic cavity are often hampered by the difficulty to orient in the endoscopic view. This is due to the small field of view and the inhomogeneous illumination, but also because abdominal organs are highly deformable and subject to complex movements. The use of flexible endoscopes further complicates these issues. In the context of a multidisciplinary project involving clinical and technical teams, we report the definition of clinical requirements and surgical workflow of abdominal endoscopic interventions, and present the design and implementation of a planning and navigation system. Some of the implemented features include: segmentation, tracking, landmark-based navigation, and combined surface and volume rendering. Our system is based on open source libraries, and is flexible and applicable to other types of interventions.

Keywords: Endoscopy · Navigation · Surgical planning · Tracking · Open source

1 Purpose

It is generally acknowledged that one of the foremost challenges of endoscopy is the difficulty to orient in the small and inhomogeneous field of view of the endoscope. The use of flexible endoscopes has led to unprecedented access to the abdominal cavity, enabling numerous procedures in a minimally invasive manner (such as natural orifice transluminal endoscopic surgery - NOTES). Conversely, the use of such flexible endoscopes, in the context of highly deformable organs exposed to constant motion, as is the case of the abdominal cavity, poses severe difficulties for the orientation and localization of target structures.

In this paper we present our work towards the development of a surgical navigation system for abdominal interventions performed using flexible endoscopes.

M. Erdt et al. (Eds.): CLIP 2013, LNCS 8361, pp. 91–98, 2014.
DOI: 10.1007/978-3-319-05666-1_12, © Springer International Publishing Switzerland 2014

In particular, Sect. 2 reports the analysis and modelling of clinical requirements and surgical workflows. Section 3 focuses on the design and implementation of the different elements of the system. This image-registered navigation system is based in electromagnetic tracking and built using open-source libraries, such as IGSTK and ITK, and it is modularized and fully extensible to cover multiple surgical applications. Section 4 shows results and Sect. 5 closes the paper with perspectives for future work.

This project is made possible by means of a close collaboration between clinical and technical teams, in a multi-disciplinary approach, focusing on the development of a practical system to be used in routine interventions.

2 Clinical Requirements and Surgical Workflow

The rationale for the system is to provide the endoscopist with the most adequate visual feedback of the location and the orientation of the endoscope, in order to improve instrument navigation and facilitating the recognition of anatomical structures. This has proven to have statistically significant benefits in enabling a better smoothness of motion [1–3].

A fundamental component of the system is a pre-operative CT scan of the subject, which is used to extract (segment) the relevant structures to the intervention, including bones, main vessels, skin, etc. As a result of these semi-automatic segmentation procedures a set of meshes are generated, which will be shown in the navigation views, to assist the endoscopist increasing their spatial awareness inside the subject.

Notice that although these segmentations are computed from the pre-operative CT, they still will provide valuable spatial context to the operator through a simulated virtual endoscopic view (automatically updated) and an "external" 3D view (handled by the operator). A set of 2D multi-planar reconstruction views provide further guidance by showing the current endoscope tip position.

The structures to be segmented depend on the protocol. For thoracic and abdominal interventions they may include bones, lungs, gallbladder, aortic trunk, celiac and superior mesenteric artery branches, kidneys and bladder, heart, trachea, and skin. The skin model of the subject is very important since it is used for the registration stage in the operating room.

Two procedures take place in the operating room: Calibration (including ICP-based registration—ICP standing for Iterative Closest Point), and Image-Guided Navigation (Fig. 1).

The workflow of the calibration phase consists of 3 steps. First, the operator launches the electromagnetic device, attaching two electromagnetic sensors (a free "pointer," and another tied to the endoscope, "endoscope sensor"). After checking that the signal level from the sensors is accurate, the patient is registered with the pointer, by touching with it a set of fiducials (anatomical landmarks). Next, a continuous tracking is performed to retrieve the anterior surface of the subject, and the application saves the locations of the "point cloud." The application computes a registration using ICP, and applies the obtained transformation to the retrieved cloud, visualizing the resulting points on top of the pre-segmented models, for the operator to decide if they match. The endoscope is activated and the operator places the

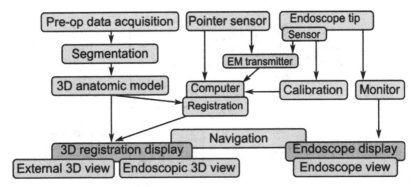

Fig. 1. Global system architecture (gray: hardware, blue: software/method, green: model/view) (Color figure online)

endoscope on top of subject's belly, and rotates the camera for the external 3D view to match the real endoscopic view/orientation with the endoscopic video to capture the relative roll of the camera. Finally, the endoscope's electromagnetic sensor fixation is calibrated with respect to the endoscope camera by touching the tip of the endoscope with the pointer.

At this moment, the endoscopic procedure and the navigation phase start (Fig. 2), the endoscopic 3D view appears, and the FOV of the endoscope is shown in the external 3D view. The application starts tracking the endoscope sensor and updates the views continuously—the operator can choose the visibility of the surface models shown in the virtual views, the MPRs in the External 3D view, and can manipulate the camera for the External 3D view at their convenience.

3   System Design and Implementation

In this section we describe technical aspects of the image-guided support system we are developing to aid during the endoscopy navigation. It is meant to be a modular system that reuses software components as much as possible. The ultimate goal is to be able to use different kinds of input systems to aid in the interventions (for therapies, or surgeries) in the operating room, as depicted in Fig. 3. The system is implemented in C++

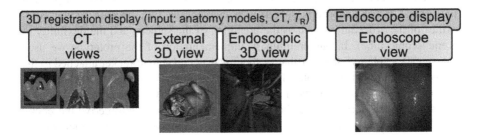

Fig. 2. The set of navigation views

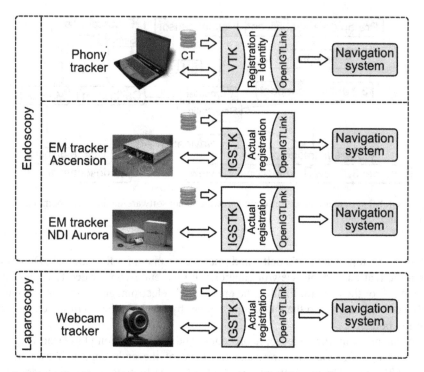

Fig. 3. General architecture of the system for a number of possible trackers and interventions

using well-known and standard open-source toolkits. The Visualization Toolkit (VTK, www.vtk.org) is used for the user interaction and visualization purposes (rendering in the 2D and 3D views, annotations, and performing volume rendering). In addition, it provides methods for manipulation of points, meshes and images, including the ICP algorithm that we have employed to align the data. Communication between devices (concretely, between the EM tracker and the navigation application) is built on top of the IGSTK toolkit (www.igstk.org), a high-level, component-based framework which provides a common functionality for image-guided surgery application. Finally, we also use OpenIGTLink (www.openigtlink.org), an open network interface for image guided therapy, to send data to the navigation part of the system.

We are currently tackling endoscopy-based procedures, such as NOTES (natural orifice transluminal endoscopy surgery)—a challenging task because of the complexities of the procedures (such as the breathing of the subject, and the flexibility of the endoscopic tube). In our preliminary implementation of the prototype we used what we call a "phony" tracker (that is, there was not an actual tracker attached to the system), consisting on a simple 2D visualization viewer that uses the keyboard to navigate through the axial slices of a pre-operative image (CT)—see Fig. 4. We used the position of the cursor within the current rendered axial slice to derive the phony location of the sensor. In addition, we provided the viewer with functionalities to change the orientation of the "endoscope" (yaw, pitch and roll) by means of key

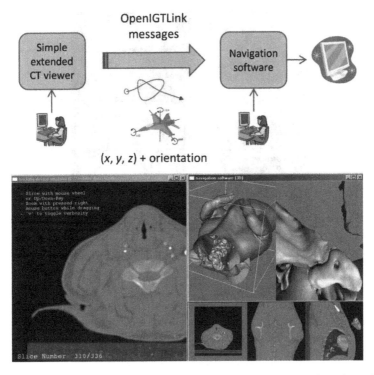

Fig. 4. Simple setting for the "phony" tracker (top) and their corresponding views (bottom), using a swine, including the external 3D view, the endoscope view, and the MPR views

strokes. All this information was packed and sent using OpenIGTLink messages (igtl::PositionMessage, with its methods SetPosition and SetQuaternion). There was no need of computing any kind of registration since the "phony" space and the pre-operative image were the same space, since we used the same CT. The application also incorporates the functionality to capture snapshots of the current views for reporting.

Next, we successfully incorporated a real electromagnetic device (in our case, the Ascension 3D Guidance trakSTAR[TM], Milton, VT, USA) to substitute the phony tracker. As shown in Fig. 3, since there is no need to visualize CT slices there is no dependency on VTK; instead we used IGSTK first to establish communication with the device and then to gather the readings of their sensors. This setting also required performing an actual registration between the spaces of the operating room and the pre-operative image, to send consistent data to the navigation system. The transformation was computed by using the iterative closest point (ICP) algorithm.

Additionally, we have added GPU-based volume rendering capabilities to show non-segmented structures (see Fig. 5, where bones and vessels with contrast are drawn with volume rendering in the endoscopic view) that leads to an enhanced augmented reality environment with respect to previous systems [4]. Also, during the navigation, if the endoscopist locates a new landmark of interest (for example, a lesion), the

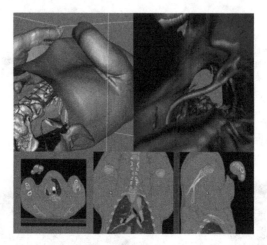

Fig. 5. Virtual navigation views using a CT scan of a swine as example—notice that volume rendering is used for the endoscopic view

software application allows tagging it for further study in the form of annotations (see Fig. 6). Finally, the system has been extended to allow storing captured poses into a file, which permits re-creating the virtual visualization for planning interventions (Fig. 7).

4   Results and Other Applications

The images above show the functionalities implemented in the current system. In addition, we have explored other uses of the navigation system, which include: cardiac

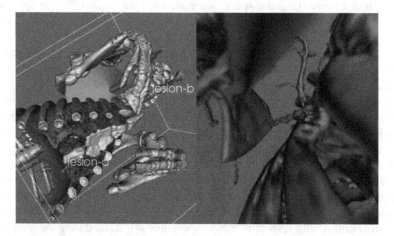

Fig. 6. 3D views with example annotations (left), and volume rendering including small vessels (right)

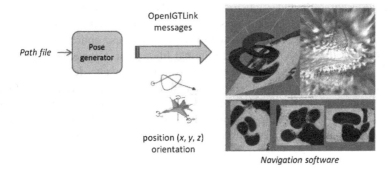

OpenIGTLink
messages

Path file

Pose
generator

position (x, y, z)
orientation

Navigation software

Fig. 7. Schema for the recreation of a path in the navigation system by using a planned path file

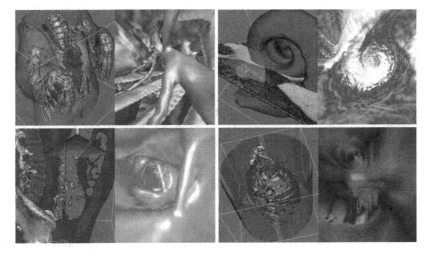

Fig. 8. Examples of usage of the navigation system: pig case, cochlear navigation, virtual colonoscopy, and virtual bronchoscopy

surgery, cochlear implantation, virtual colonoscopies and bronchoscopy, as exemplified in Fig. 8.

Our preliminary experiences show that the system is very versatile, and allows seamless integration in the surgical workflow of different surgical interventions.

5   Conclusion and Future Work

This paper has reported the design and development of a software tool for image-based navigation in endoscopic abdominal interventions. The modular system is written in C++, and is based on common and well-established open source libraries: VTK, IGSTK, OpenIGTKLink. Integration in the operating room is realised, and cases have been scheduled in order to validate the use of our system.

Work in progress includes integration with NDI Aurora electromagnetic trackers (NDI, Waterloo, Ontario, Canada), reusing most of the code and modules, as depicted in Fig. 3. Also, for laparoscopic interventions we plan to use optical trackers such as webcams (using the ArUco library—a minimal library for Augmented reality applications based on OpenCV, www.uco.es/investiga/grupos/ava/no-de/26) or the Polaris System (also by NDI) to derive the location and pose of the surgery tools within the patient—again sharing most of the code. We also plan to improve and validate the navigation system using Lego phantoms along the lines of the Image-Guided tutorial [5], and perform its actual integration in the in the operating room.

References

1. Fernández-Esparrach, G., San José Estépar, R., Guarner-Argente, C., Martínez-Pallí, G., Navarro, R., Rodríguez de Miguel, C., Córdova, H., Thompson, C.C., Lacy, A.M., Donoso, L., Ayuso-Colella, J.R., Ginès, A., Pellisé, M., Llach, J., Vosburgh, K.G.: The role of a computed tomography-based image registered navigation system for natural orifice transluminal endoscopic surgery: a comparative study in a porcine model. Endoscopy **42**(12), 1096–1103 (2010)
2. Córdova, H., San José Estépar, R., Rodríguez-D'Jesús, A., Martínez-Pallí, G., Arguis, P., Rodríguez de Miguel, C., Navarro-Ripoll, R., Perdomo, J.M., Cuatrecasas, M., Llach, J., Vosburgh, K.G., Fernández-Esparrach, G.: Comparative study of NOTES alone versus NOTES guided by a new image registration system for navigation in the mediastinum: a study in a porcine model. Gastrointest. Endosc. **77**(1), 102–107 (2013)
3. Azagury, D.E., Ryou, M., Shaikh, S.N., San José Estépar, R., Lengyel, B.I., Jagadeesan, J., Vosburgh, K.G., Thompson, C.C.: Real-time computed tomography-based augmented reality for natural orifice transluminal endoscopic surgery navigation. Br. J. Surg. **99**(9), 1246–1253 (2012)
4. San José Estépar, R., Stylopoulos, N., Ellis, R., Samset, E., Westin, C.-F., Thompson, C., Vosburgh, K.: Towards scarless surgery: an endoscopic ultrasound navigation system for transgastric access procedures. Comput. Aided Surg. **12**(6), 311–324 (2007)
5. Güler, Ö, Yaniv, Z.: Image-Guided Interventions Tutorial using the Image-Guided Surgery Toolkit. http://isiswiki.georgetown.edu/zivy/igiTutorial/igiTutorial.html

Automatic Optimization of Depth Electrode Trajectory Planning

Rina Zelmann[✉], Silvain Beriault, Kelvin Mok, Claire Haegelen,
Jeff Hall, G. Bruce Pike, Andre Olivier, and D. Louis Collins

Neurology and Neurosurgery, Montreal Neurological Institute,
Montreal, QC, Canada
rina.zelmann@mail.mcgill.ca

Abstract. This paper presents a fully automatic procedure for optimization of depth electrode implantation planning in epilepsy. To record intracranial EEG in some patients with intractable epilepsy, depth electrodes are implanted through holes in the skull. The proposed fully automatic procedure maximizes recording coverage of the target volume by estimating the EEG recorded from each contact, while minimizing the risk of approaching vessels and other critical structures. All structures, including the hippocampus and amygdala were automatically segmented. We retrospectively validated the procedure for mesial temporal lobe implantations in 11 hemispheres. The automatic trajectories recorded from a larger volume of interest than the original manually selected trajectories while better avoiding the segmented structures. The procedure is integrated into a neuronavigation system enabling the surgeon to visualize the selected trajectories from an ordered list and, if necessary, enables re-planning a trajectory in near real time.

Keywords: Depth electrode implantation · Trajectory optimization · EEG recording maximization · Automatic target segmentation · Image guided neurosurgery

1 Introduction

Epilepsy affects 5–6/1000 of the population, 30 % of whom are refractory to medication. Mesial temporal lobe epilepsy is the most common type of refractory epilepsy, accounting for 70 % of the cases [1]. Some of these patients are candidates for surgery which, when successful, leads to seizure freedom. As part of the pre-surgical evaluation, intracranial EEG is sometimes recorded to precisely localize the region responsible of seizure generation. Multiple depth electrodes are surgically implanted through holes in the skull, each with 8–10 equally spaced contacts. Current implantation planning strategy consists of visual inspection of the patient's MRI (with segmented vessels) to manually search for a path that reaches the target while avoiding vessels. The procedure is time-consuming, potentially error prone and suboptimal as the location of each contact is not considered. Considering the precise contact location is paramount to accurately identify the epileptic focus based on intracranial EEG.

M. Erdt et al. (Eds.): CLIP 2013, LNCS 8361, pp. 99–107, 2014.
DOI: 10.1007/978-3-319-05666-1_13, © Springer International Publishing Switzerland 2014

Automatic trajectory planning in minimally invasive neurosurgery is an area of active research, in particular for deep brain stimulation (DBS) [2–5] and abdominal surgery (e.g. [6]). In these frameworks the optimal trajectory is obtained by minimizing the risk of passing through vessels or other relevant structures. Importantly in [2, 3] a list of trajectories, ordered in terms of risk, enables the surgeon to select the most suitable trajectory during the intervention. Specifically for epilepsy, De Momi presented a procedure that considers the optimization of multiple electrodes [7]. Target and entry points were visually identified and search spaces defined as a sphere around these points. As in the case of DBS, optimization only considered minimizing risk. In all these cases, the target is a point visually defined by the surgeon or it is obtained based on atlas [4]. While this approach is reasonable for DBS, the goal of depth electrode implantation in epilepsy is to maximally record EEG from a given *volume* (e.g. hippocampus). Thus, optimal placement of electrodes to maximize coverage of the region of interest is important, but has not been addressed.

In some patients with a suspected mesial temporal focus the question is whether the seizures originate from the hippocampus (HC), the amygdala (AG) or the temporal neocortex. Thus, it is important not only to accurately record from deep structures, but also to obtain good coverage of the surrounding neocortex. Although electrodes are implanted through the temporal neocortex and EEG recordings analyzed, with manual planning it is not feasible to consider each contact's location during planning.

In this study, we propose a novel fully automatic planning procedure that maximizes recording from the volume of interest and surrounding gray matter, while constraining trajectories to safe paths. To this end, we modeled each trajectory as a cylinder, estimated the recording capability of individual contacts, automatically segmented MRI data, and computed a final score by aggregating a weighted set of surgical constraints. To allow its clinical use during surgery, the automatically generated trajectory list, ordered in terms of an aggregated score based on estimated risks and recording volumes, is integrated into a locally developed neuronavigation system [8].

2 Methods

2.1 Patient Selection and Electrode Information

Six patients with medically intractable epilepsy and a presumed temporal generator, had depth electrodes implanted in the mesial temporal lobe, a pre-implantation MRI with gadolinium injection that allowed for vessel segmentation, and an MRI immediately after depth electrodes explantation that allowed for the identification of the electrode's position after the investigation. MRIs could not be obtained during the invasive investigation because of electrode-MRI incompatibility. Five patients had bilateral implantation. We considered each hemisphere independently for a total of 11 hemispheres and a grand total of 27 electrodes. All patients gave informed consent in agreement with the Research Ethics Board of our center.

Each electrode had a diameter of 0.4 mm and comprised nine contacts (surface area 0.8 mm^2) separated by 5 mm. The deepest contact consisted of the tip of the steel core stripped of insulation. This contact had a length of 1 mm, while all other contacts were formed from stripped sections of the marginal wire to create 0.5 mm long coils.

2.2 MRI Acquisition and Image Processing

Acquisition and Pre-processing. Pre-implantation, before (T1w-Pre) and after gadolinium injection (T1w-Gd), and post-explantation (T1w-Post) clinical MRIs were acquired on a clinical 1.5 Tesla GE Signa EXCITE (General Electric, Milwaukee, WI, USA) with T1-weighted sequences (180 slices, 0.5 × 0.5 × 1 mm resolution, TE = 8 ms, TR = 23 ms, flip angle 20°). Image intensity non-uniformity was corrected (N3 default parameters; [9]), followed by linear image intensity normalization [10] and non-rigid transformation to the ICBM152 model [11]. A patient-specific brain mask was created (BEaST; [12]). T1w-Gd and T1w-Post were rigidly registered to T1w-Pre.

Segmentation of Critical Structures. AG and HC (the target structures) were segmented on the pre-processed T1w-Pre, with a fully automated method based on a template library and label fusion [13] (Fig. 1A). Segmentations were visually validated by an expert neurosurgeon. The HC was divided in anterior and posterior sections at the plane perpendicular to the main axis at its centroid since independent electrodes are aimed at each section. T1w-Pre was processed with tissue classification [14] to segment gray matter (GM), white matter, ventricles, and the different lobes. In particular, GM in the temporal lobe (Fig. 1B) and sulci patterns were extracted. Angiographic data (T1w-Gd) was rescaled to 0.5 mm isotropic resolution, denoised with a non local means filter [15], and processed with Frangi's 3D multi-scale vesselness filter [16]. This filter is sensitive to tubular structures and returns a voxel likelihood [0.0–1.0] of blood vessel presence (Fig. 1C). To compare the automatic trajectories with the original implantations, implanted electrodes were segmented by visually localizing the tracks on T1w-Post (Fig. 1D).

2.3 Surgical Constraints for Optimization

Optimization was performed in three steps. First, trajectories intersecting vessels or the ventricles were rejected. Second, the risk with respect to the constraints detailed below was computed. Finally, the "reward" of recording from a large volume in the

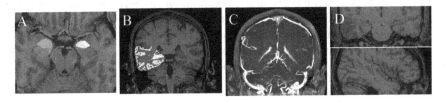

Fig. 1. Segmented critical structures and true implanted electrode in patient 3. (A) Automatically segmented HC and AG overlaid on T1w-Pre. (B) Automatically segmented GM of the left temporal lobe on T1w-Pre. (C) Vessels obtained from T1w-Gd. (D) Visually segmented true implanted electrodes on T1w-Post. In blue, electrode targeting the anterior HC (Color figure online).

target structures and surrounding GM was computed. Trajectories were constrained to safe paths by minimizing these constraints:

1. *Avoidance of blood vessels.* Summed and maximum distance to vessels was maximized. Vessel avoidance is the major surgical constraint.
2. *Avoidance of sulci.* Trajectories that may cross a sulcus were discarded. Distance from sulci was maximized since small vessels may lie at the fundus of the sulcus.
3. *Avoidance of lateral ventricle.* This constraint is particularly important for trajectories targeting the anterior HC, since the lateral ventricles should be avoided. Trajectories that were too close to the ventricles were discarded.
4. *Avoidance of other electrodes.* We checked that the cohort of best trajectories did not cross. If so, the best cohort without overlap was chosen.

The volume recorded was maximized by integrating the recordings from each contact on the following structures:

5. *Recording of Target Volume.* In depth electrode implantations with a suspected mesial temporal generator, three targets are of interest: AG, anterior HC and posterior HC. We maximized the combined coverage from contacts within them.
6. *Recording of Gray Matter.* Only the first 2 or 3 contacts of each electrode are implanted within the target. Remaining contacts are useful to record from surrounding GM, to understand seizure propagation or to differentiate between pure temporal and neocortical epilepsy. We maximized the recording from each contact in GM.

2.4   Automatic Depth Electrode Trajectory Planning

The trajectory planning algorithm maximizes the recorded EEG by considering the contacts that lie within the structure of interest, while constraining to safe trajectories. Possible entry points defining the allowed search space were selected once by the head of the neuronavigation unit on the left temporal lobe of the ICBM152 model by identifying a broad possible region of entry (e.g. secondary temporal gyrus for anterior HC). These areas were warped to each hemisphere's surface. Target search spaces were obtained from the segmented deep structures. One thousand possible trajectories were uniformly randomly selected for evaluation by the algorithm.

Let $tr_i(ep, tp)$ be each possible trajectory, with ep an entry point and tp a target point. Each tr_i is modeled as a central line (the electrode) where the contacts are located surrounded by a cylinder of radius 5 mm, since being at 5 mm or further away from a critical structure could be considered of equivalent risk. The risk score (negative score, $f_{neg}(tr_i)$) is similar to the one proposed in [2]. It is defined as the aggregation of all possible risks:

$$f_{neg}(tr_i) = \sum_j [w_{max}^j . risk_{max}(tr_i, j) + w_{sum}^j . risk_{sum}(tr_i, j)] \qquad (1)$$

where $risk_{max}(tr_i, j)$ is the maximum encountered risk and $risk_{sum}(tr_i, j)$ is the sum of all risks along each trajectory, weighted by the distance to the center of the cylinder.

W^j_{max} and w^j_{sum} are the weights for each of the j surgical constraints described in the previous section ($w^{vessel}_{max} = 0.6$, $w^{vessel}_{sum} = 0.3$, $w^{sulci}_{max} = 0.5$, $w^{ventr}_{max} = 0.5$). Weights were defined together with the neurosurgeons and then normalized to sum one.

The risk was computed based on the trajectory since it is important to avoid critical structures along the implantation. On the other hand, the reward score (positive score, $f_{pos}(tr_i)$) was computed based on the EEG that can be recorded by each contact of the electrode within the volume of interest. The volume recorded by a particular contact was estimated to decay as the square of the distance from the center of the contact. The distance map from the edges of each structure was computed [17]. We integrated the structure's distance map with the combined recording volume of the electrode. In this way we considered that it is more relevant to record from the center of the target, but even more so to record with multiple contacts. Figure 2 illustrates this method.

To understand seizure propagation, not only optimizing coverage of the target is important, but also recording from the surrounding neocortex. Thus, the reward score is the weighted sum of volume recorded ($recVol_k$) from the target and temporal GM:

$$f_{pos}(tr_i) = w_{target} \cdot recVol_{target}(tr_i) + w_{GM} \cdot recVol_{GM}(tr_i) \tag{2}$$

where w_{target} is the weight corresponding to recording from the target and w_{GM} corresponds to recording from GM in the temporal lobe ($w_{target} = 0.8$, $w_{GM} = 0.2$).

A list of trajectories was than obtained by ordering the cost function $F(tr_i)$, which aggregates risk ($w_{neg} = 0.75$) and reward ($w_{pos} = 0.25$) scores:

$$F(tr_i) = w_{pos}(1 - f_{pos}(tr_i)) + w_{neg} \cdot f_{neg}(tr_i) \tag{3}$$

The procedure was integrated into a locally developed neuronavigation system (IBIS; [8]). The list of ordered trajectories is presented to the surgeons to visualize trajectories overlaid on the MRI images. Segmented structures were included. The best cohort of trajectories (AG, anterior HC and posterior HC) was checked to avoid crossing of electrodes (min distance: 5 mm). Thus, the best 3-electrode cohort had the smallest combined score out of the non-intersecting trajectories. Weights could be modified in the GUI, which updates scores and trajectory order.

Fig. 2. (A) Estimation of recording from each electrode's contact in axial view. (B) Distance map of anterior HC in hemisphere 9. (C) Overlay of A and B indicating recording region.

2.5   Validation

Since this is a retrospective study, we quantitatively compared the best cohort of fully automatic trajectories to the true implanted trajectories. To this end, the original trajectories, obtained from electrodes segmented on T1w-Post, were scored using the same cost function described above. Wilcoxon test was used for statistical comparison. Significance level was set at $p < 0.01$. In addition, to evaluate clinical feasibility, as a 2nd validation, the head of the neuronavigation unit qualitatively evaluated if trajectories in the best cohort could be clinically used in reality. This was visually reviewed in a similar way as in the operating room: navigating in 3D (with brain surface, vessels and segmented targets), bird's eye view, trajectory view, and 2D views.

3   Results

We compared a total of 27 trajectories in 11 hemispheres. The automatic trajectories recorded from a significantly larger target volume ($p < 0.01$) and from more temporal GM ($p < 0.001$) than the original manual trajectories, while staying significantly further away from segmented vessels (median minimum distance AUTO = 4.03 mm, MANUAL = 1.59 mm; $p < 0.01$). Figure 3 shows box plots for volume recorded and vessel comparisons.

Figure 4 shows an example of automatic trajectories for the three structures and the avoidance of vessels in hemisphere 9. This and the next figure show typical examples.

Figure 5 shows a comparison of automatic and manual trajectories in hemisphere 10. In particular the zoom in Fig. 5B illustrates that the automatic trajectory finds a target closer to the center of the AG volume than the original manual trajectory. Thus, the EEG recordings are likely to represent a better sampling of AG activity.

The qualitative validation showed that 25/27 trajectories (92.5 %) satisfied the proposed surgical constraints and were feasible from a clinical stand point. For the 2 rejected trajectories, others in the list were also inspected and found suitable.

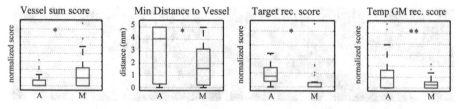

Fig. 3. Box plots comparing automatic and manual trajectories for all 27 trajectories pooled together. In each plot: *left* automatic (A), *right* manual (M) plan. (A) Sum score for vessels risk. (B) Minimum distance to vessel. (C) Recorded target volume. (D) Recorded temporal GM. Significant difference was found in all comparisons (* indicates $p < 0.01$; ** indicates $p < 0.001$).

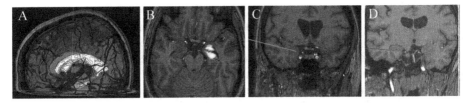

Fig. 4. Example of automatically optimized trajectories aiming at the AG (blue), anterior HC (magenta) and posterior HC (orange) in hemisphere 9. (A) 3D view with vessels. (B) Axial view showing the target for AG and anterior HC. (C) Trajectory view for AG and (D) anterior HC (Color figure online).

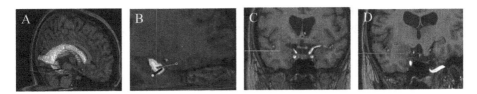

Fig. 5. Example of an automatic and the original manual trajectory in hemisphere 10. (A) 3D view with all electrodes. Original plans are shown in green, automatic plans in cyan. (B) Automatic and the manual target for the AG (displayed with AG distance map). Note that the automatic target reaches the center. (C) Trajectory view of manual and (D) automatic plans for AG.

Processing time was 2 min per hemisphere. This step is processed prior to surgery, and thus it is not critical. Re-estimation of best trajectories (by modifying the weights) took less than 1 s. By dividing the procedure in a pre-surgical processing used for planning and allowing for a rapid modification of the surgical weights in almost real time in the operation room, our system could be useful for planning before surgery and for adjusting the trajectories during depth electrode surgical implantations.

4 Discussion

In this study, we presented a computer assisted procedure that automatically optimizes trajectories for depth electrode implantation in mesial temporal structures. This procedure is the first to maximize the recording volume by modeling the contribution of each contact, while maximizing avoidance of critical structures. Our analysis is fully automatic, from the segmentation of the volume of interest to the optimization of the trajectories. A list of ordered trajectories is presented, enabling surgeons to select the best cohort before implantation, validate trajectories during surgery and, if necessary, re-plan in near real time. Based on the same clinical data, we showed that the automatic procedure is safer and records more information than the original manual trajectories. However, this validation was based on the same assumptions and segmented tissue used for the automatic method. Even though these assumptions were discussed with the neurosurgeons and could therefore be considered similar for automatic and manual planning, they could have biased the validation. Errors in the segmentation could be another source of bias. The qualitative confirmation by an expert indicates that the procedure could be useful for clinical use. Future development includes implementing a margin of uncertainty to account for inaccuracy in segmentation, prospective evaluation of the procedure during planning and intervention and implementation to implantation in other regions, considering particular constraints.

In summary, the presented automatic procedure increases the accuracy and the amount of information obtained with implanted depth electrodes while reducing the risk of crossing critical structures comparing to manual planning. This procedure will improve the outcome of invasive investigation of patients with refractory epilepsy, leading to better surgical planning and patient outcomes.

Acknowledgements. This study was supported in part by CIHR MOP-97820 and by MNI CIBC postdoctoral fellowship in brain imaging.

References

1. Engel, J., Pedley, T.A.: Epilepsy: A Comprehensive Textbook. Wolters Kluwer Health/ Lippincott Williams & Wilkins, Philadelphia (2008)
2. Bériault, S., Subaie, F.A., Lalys, F., Collins, D.L., Pike, G.B., Sadikot, A.F.: A multi-modal approach to computer-assisted deep brain stimulation trajectory planning. Int. J. Comput. Assist. Radiol. Surg. **7**, 1–18 (2012)
3. Essert, C., Haegelen, C., Lalys, F., Abadie, A., Jannin, P.: Automatic computation of electrode trajectories for deep brain stimulation: a hybrid symbolic and numerical approach. Int. J. Comput. Assist. Radiol. Surg. **7**, 517–532 (2012)
4. Guo, T., Parrent, A.G., Peters, T.M.: Automatic target and trajectory identification for deep brain stimulation (DBS) procedures. In: Ayache, Nicholas, Ourselin, Sébastien, Maeder, Anthony (eds.) MICCAI 2007, Part I. LNCS, vol. 4791, pp. 483–490. Springer, Heidelberg (2007)
5. Liu, Y., et al.: A surgeon specific automatic path planning algorithm for deep brain stimulation. In: Proceedings of the SPIE 8316 Medical Imaging 2011, p. 83161D (2011)
6. Seitel, A., et al.: Computer-assisted trajectory planning for percutaneous needle insertions. Med. Phys. **38**, 3246–3259 (2011)
7. De Momi, E., Caborni, C., Cardinale, F., Castana, L., Casaceli, G., Cossu, M., Antiga, L., Ferrigno, G.: Automatic trajectory planner for StereoElectroEncephaloGraphy procedures: a retrospective study. IEEE Trans. Biomed. Eng. **4**, 986–993 (2013)
8. Mercier, L., et al.: New prototype neuronavigation system based on preoperative imaging and intraoperative freehand ultrasound: system description and validation. Int. J. Comput. Assist. Radiol. Surg. **6**, 507–522 (2011)
9. Sled, J.G., Zijdenbos, A.P., Evans, A.C.: A nonparametric method for automatic correction of intensity nonuniformity in MRI data. IEEE Trans. Med. Imaging **17**(1), 87–97 (1998)
10. Nyul, L.G., Udupa, J.K., Saha, P.K.: Incorporating a measure of local scale in voxel-based 3-D image registration. IEEE Trans. Med. Imaging **22**, 228–237 (2003)
11. Mazziotta, J., Toga, A., Evans, A., Fox, P., Lancaster, J., Zilles, K., et al.: A probabilistic atlas and reference system for the human brain: international consortium for brain mapping (ICBM). Philos. Trans. R. Soc. Lond. B Biol. Sci. **356**, 1293–1322 (2001)

12. Eskildsen, S.F.: BEaST: brain extraction based on nonlocal segmentation technique. NeuroImage **59**, 2362–2373 (2012)
13. Collins, D.L., Pruessner, J.C.: Towards accurate, automatic segmentation of the hippocampus and amygdala from MRI by augmenting ANIMAL with a template library and label fusion. NeuroImage **52**, 1355–1366 (2010)
14. Collins, D.L., Zijdenbos, A., Baaré, W., Evans, A.: ANIMAL+INSECT: improved cortical structure segmentation. In: Kuba, A., Šáamal, M., Todd-Pokropek, A. (eds.) IPMI 1999. LNCS, vol. 1613, pp. 210–223. Springer, Heidelberg (1999)
15. Coupé, P., Yger, P., Prima, S., Hellier, P., Kervrann, C., Barillot, C.: An optimized blockwise nonlocal means denoising filter for 3-D magnetic resonance images. IEEE Trans. Med. Imaging **27**, 425–441 (2008)
16. Frangi, A.F., Niessen, W.J., Vincken, K.L., Viergever, M.A.: Multiscale vessel enhancement filtering. In: Wells, W.M., Colchester, A.C.F., Delp, S.L. (eds.) MICCAI 1998. LNCS, vol. 1496, pp. 130–137. Springer, Heidelberg (1998)
17. Danielsson, P.E.: Euclidean distance mapping. Comput. Graph. Image Process. **14**, 227–248 (1980)

Towards a Clinical Stereoscopic Augmented Reality System for Laparoscopic Surgery

Xin Kang, Jihun Oh, Emmanuel Wilson, Ziv Yaniv,
Timothy D. Kane, Craig A. Peters, and Raj Shekhar$^{(\boxtimes)}$

Sheikh Zayed Institute for Pediatric Surgical Innovation, Children's National
Medical Center, Washington, DC, USA
{xkang, jhoh, ewilson, zyaniv, tkane, crpeters,
rshekhar}@cnmc.org

Abstract. We describe our development of a complete real-time stereoscopic augmented reality system that overlays laparoscopic ultrasound (LUS) images on stereoscopic laparoscopic video for conventional laparoscopic surgery. The system was designed and developed to achieve near-term clinical evaluation as a primary goal. Special consideration was paid to system interactivity, accuracy and easy integration within the existing clinical workflow. Custom-designed fixtures for the two imaging devices were created to avoid their recalibration in the operating room and thus to minimize setup time. The system was assembled on a rolling cart to make it portable for the use in the operating room. Utilizing our optimized design and hardware-accelerated implementation, the system achieved a low system latency of approximately 150 ms. The LUS image-to-video registration accuracy, measured in terms of target registration accuracy and recorded separately for the left and right eye channels of the stereoscopic camera, was 3.34±0.59 mm and 2.76±0.68 mm.

Keywords: Stereoscopic augmented reality (AR) · Real-time AR · Clinical prototype · Laparoscopic surgery

1 Introduction

In minimally invasive laparoscopic surgery, the laparoscopic camera is currently the primary means to provide real-time visual information on the surgical field. However, conventional laparoscopes have two significant limitations. First, they provide only a flat 2D representation of the 3D surgical field, introducing ambiguity in depth perception. Second, they are incapable of providing information on internal structures and cannot visualize surgical targets located beneath the exposed organ surfaces.

Several research groups have developed systems and methods to provide combined surface and internal anatomy information by overlaying pre- and intra-operative tomographic images on the laparoscopic video. These augmented reality (AR) efforts have been reported for both robotic surgery [1, 2] and conventional surgery [3–7].

The systems and methods using pre- and intra-operative CT and MR images have many limitations that make them less robust and reliable and thus less desirable for operating room (OR) use. These limitations arise from (1) the inability of

M. Erdt et al. (Eds.): CLIP 2013, LNCS 8361, pp. 108–116, 2014.
DOI: 10.1007/978-3-319-05666-1_14, © Springer International Publishing Switzerland 2014

pre-operative imaging to properly and accurately describe the ever-deforming anatomy during surgery, (2) the fact that the currently employed registration procedures are mostly rigid when the soft-tissue organs deform non-rigidly throughout the surgery; and (3) the subjective and non-reproducible accuracy of manual or semi-automatic registration.

For continuous and automatic updates of the surgical field, Shekhar et al. [7] acquired low-dose non-contrast CT continuously throughout a surgical procedure. The investigators also acquired a standard contrast CT scan immediately before starting surgery. Applying high-speed deformable registration, the vasculature data was transferred from the initial contrast CT to intra-operative non-contrast CT. Although the method does track continuous deformation of the surgical anatomy and provides accurate CT-to-video registration, the risk of high radiation exposure to the patient and the surgical team renders this approach clinically impractical in the foreseeable future.

Laparoscopic ultrasound (LUS) can provide real-time intra-operative images without any ionizing radiation. An advantage of using LUS in combination with live laparoscopic video is that soft-tissue deformation does not need to be modeled, and accurate image-to-video registration can be achieved with standard tracking techniques. Leven et al. [1] took this approach to create a module for the da Vinci robotic surgical system (Intuitive Surgical, Sunnyvale, CA) that superimposes LUS images on stereoscopic laparoscopic video. The rigid LUS probe is tracked by means of a vision-based method that localizes a distinctive pattern situated close to the LUS transducer.

Cheung et al. [3] have developed a platform that uses a stereoscopic laparoscope and a flexible-tip LUS. The two devices were tracked using an electromagnetic (EM) tracking system. The wired EM sensors were affixed to the LUS transducer and the laparoscope. A phantom study was performed to mimic minimally invasive partial nephrectomy [4] in the laboratory. The platform may not be suitable for clinical use since it was designed mainly for feasibility study and its usability was not reported.

In this paper, we describe our development of a complete stereoscopic AR system for conventional laparoscopic surgery. The system overlays LUS images on stereo laparoscopic video in real time. Unlike prior developments that were limited to research prototypes and laboratory testing, our system has been designed and developed by a team of biomedical engineers and minimally invasive surgeons with near-term clinical demonstration as a primary goal. Tested thus far in the laboratory and in animal studies, the system offers acceptable accuracy, low latency, minimal setup time, and minimal changes to the existing surgical workflow for clinical use.

2   Method

2.1   System Design

Our stereoscopic AR system uses two FDA-approved imaging devices: a vision system (VSII, Visionsense Corp., New York, NY) with a stereo laparoscope and an LUS scanner (flex Focus 700, BK Medical, Herlev, Denmark). The stereo laparoscope has a 70-degree field of view, a fixed focal length of 2.95 mm, and an interpupillary distance (IPD) of 1.04 mm. It further features an integrated light source and automatic white balance. The LUS transducer has an operating frequency range from 5 MHz to 10 MHz with a maximum allowable scan depth of 13 cm. The LUS system is capable of gray-scale B-mode and color Doppler mode scanning. An optical tracker (Polaris, Northern Digital Inc., Waterloo, Canada) is used to track the pose (location and orientation) of the stereo laparoscope and the LUS transducer in real time.

Utilizing the optical tracking data, the LUS images are registered and then overlaid on the stereoscopic video through hardware-accelerated image processing and image fusion. Consequently, two ultrasound-augmented video streams, one for the left eye and the other for the right eye, are generated. Finally, the composite AR streams are rendered for interlaced 3D display. These functions were accomplished in the fusion module. Figure 1 depicts the architecture of this module. The module is implemented on a 64-bit Windows 7 PC with an 8-core 3.2 GHz Intel CPU, 12 GB memory, and an NVidia Quadro 4000 graphics card.

To acquire images from the two imaging devices in a fast manner, the stereoscopic video and LUS images are streamed to the fusion module over gigabyte Ethernet from the two imaging devices. A custom software library, based on OEM Ethernet communication protocol, was developed to communicate with the LUS scanner. Using this library, our system can fetch LUS images and query imaging parameters (image size, pixel size, imaging mode, and imaging depth). Stereoscopic video images are similarly streamed from the vision system using its Ethernet OEM interface.

2.2   System Calibration

For a successful clinical AR system, the two types of images must be spatially registered with sufficient accuracy. This necessitates accurate calibration of the two imaging devices because any calibration errors will lead to misalignment in the stereoscopic AR visualization.

For stereo laparoscope calibration, a custom-designed calibration phantom was used. It consists of a checkerboard of alternating 5-mm black and white squares in the central region surrounded by a border that is 1 mm higher than the central region (Fig. 2). Four divots (in red and green in Fig. 2) with a depth of 1 mm were created near the four corners of the border. The size of the squares was chosen to ensure that the entire checkerboard stayed within the stereo laparoscope's field of view at the

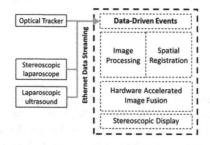

Fig. 1. Architecture of the fusion module.

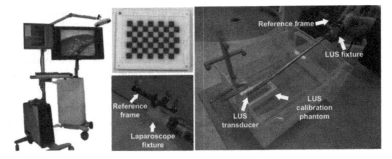

Fig. 2. The system on a rolling cart, the camera calibration phantom, the ultrasound calibration phantom and the custom-designed fixtures for optical tracking (Color figure online).

working distance of 5 cm–10 cm. The phantom was printed using a 3D printer (Objet500 Connex, Stratasys, Eden Prairie, MN) with sub-millimeter accuracy. The method proposed by Zhang [8] was used for intrinsic parameters estimation. The transformation from the laparoscope to the reference frame attached to it was determined from the coordinates of the corners of the checkerboard. By locating the four divots using a tracked stylus, the locations of the checkerboard corners with respect to the reference frame were determined. Furthermore, although the laparoscope can be treated as a stereoscopic camera pair, it was treated as two standalone cameras, each of which was calibrated separately.

For LUS calibration, we extended the ultrasound imaging research library PLUS [9] by incorporating our data streaming library. Thus, streamed LUS images rather than screenshots of the scanner display formed the input for calibration. A calibration phantom with known geometry for PLUS was 3D printed with sub-millimeter accuracy. Two wires forming two "N" shapes (called N-wires) with known geometry related to the phantom reference frame were made. The intersecting points of the two N-wires with the LUS imaging plane were used for calibration. We used 0.2 mm suturing wires since it produced clear intersecting points with little artifacts in the LUS images.

2.3 Easy Setup for Clinical Use

To track the stereo laparoscope and the LUS transducer optically, reference frames with reflective spheres need to be affixed on them. Because sterilization must precede OR use, an easy mechanism to detach the reference frames from the imaging devices and then re-attach in the OR is desirable. System calibration could be repeated in the OR after re-attaching the reference frames, however, doing so would consume expensive OR time and require an extra technician in the surgical team.

We avoid performing calibration in the OR by re-using laboratory calibration results. This is achieved using our custom-designed mechanical fixtures (see Fig. 2) that are attached to the stereo laparoscope and the LUS transducer uniquely and serve as mounts for the reference frames. In this manner, the reference frames are connected to the devices in exactly the same position as they were before dismounting. This strategy maintains a fixed geometric relationship between the reference frames (and reflecting markers) and the imaging devices before and after sterilization. The fixture for the stereo laparoscope was printed on a 3D printer and made of a synthetic resin. The fixture for the LUS transducer was machined from an aluminum alloy. Both fixtures can withstand the standard sterilization process.

To make the system portable for OR use, all the components were assembled on a custom-designed rolling cart with an articulated arm for mounting the optical tracker.

3   Experiments and Results

3.1   System Latency

The processing time of the fusion module was measured by imaging a high-resolution digital clock. The difference between the actual time and the time seen in the output image of our fusion module is the processing latency. Note that this measurement included the time of streaming video data from the vision system. The fusion module ran in full-operation mode when measuring the processing latency. The processing latency was 144±19 ms. Independently, we also estimated the latency of streaming LUS images using PLUS and found it to be 230±12 ms.

3.2   System Accuracy

The LUS image-to-video registration accuracy and calibration accuracies of the two imaging devices were measured. The standard target registration error (TRE) metric was used to quantify these accuracies. To measure the LUS image-to-video registration TRE, a target point was imaged using the LUS and its pixel location was identified in the overlaid LUS images. Aiming the laparoscope to the target point from different viewpoints, the 3D location of the target point was calculated using triangulation and compared with its actual location obtained from a tracked pointer. In our experiments, the LUS image-to-video registration TREs were 3.34±0.59 mm and 2.76±0.68 mm for the left- and right-eye channels, respectively.

For the stereo laparoscope calibration TRE, images of the calibration pattern were acquired from different viewpoints. Then, the 3D location of the pattern corners were computed using triangulation and compared with their actual locations. Treating the stereo laparoscope as two standalone cameras, the calibration TREs were 0.93±0.18 mm and 0.93±0.19 mm for the left- and right-eye channels, respectively.

For the LUS calibration TRE, a target point was imaged using the LUS. Its 3D location was estimated using the calibration result and compared with the actual location obtained from a tracked pointer. The TRE of the LUS calibration was 1.51±0.39 mm. The error was larger than what is previously reported in the literature using PLUS. This is mainly due to the long shaft of the LUS (Fig. 2). The distance from the reference frame to the LUS transducer is approximately 287 mm. This is considerably larger when compared to non-laparoscopic probes.

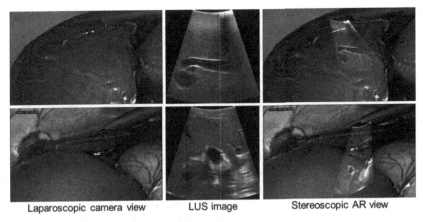

Laparoscopic camera view   LUS image   Stereoscopic AR view

Fig. 3. Two stereoscopic AR video snapshots (left-eye channel) recorded during the phantom (top) and animal (bottom) studies. Each row shows the original stereo laparoscopic camera image (left column), the original LUS image (middle column), and the stereoscopic AR image generated by our system (right column).

3.3   Phantom and Animal Studies

The system was tested in a phantom study and two animal studies involving swine. In the phantom study, an intraoperative abdominal ultrasound phantom (IOUSFAN, Kyoto Kagaku Co. Ltd., Kyoto, Japan), created specifically for laparoscopic applications, was used. It includes realistic models of the liver, spleen, kidneys, pancreas, biliary tract, and detailed vascular structures, and simulated lesions such as biliary stones cysts, and solid tumors. A stereoscopic AR video snapshot (left-eye channel) recorded during the phantom study is shown in the top row of Fig. 3.

The animal studies were performed on two 40-kg Yorkshire swine by minimally invasive laparoscopic surgeons. Using the stereoscopic AR system, right kidney, liver, and biliary structures were examined by the surgeons with the real-time LUS images superimposed on the stereo laparoscopic video to provide internal anatomical details of the organs. Stereoscopic AR video snapshots (left-eye channel) recorded during the animal studies are shown in the bottom row of Fig. 3.

4   Discussion

Developing an AR system ready for clinical evaluation requires that the system be interactive, accurate, and integrate easily within the existing clinical workflow. In the present work, in addition to carrying out technical development, we paid considerable attentions to these design criteria and obtained acceptable performance for each.

The processing time including stereoscopic video streaming and stereoscopic AR processing was approximately 144 ms. This low latency comes from optimized system design and hardware-accelerated implementation. In our system, data streaming via Ethernet OEM interfaces significantly reduced communication overhead. Additionally, texture mapping, alpha blending and interlaced display were performed using

OpenGL on a quad-buffered graphics processing unit (GPU), which significantly reduced the AR processing time. As for the latency of LUS image streaming, our experiments attribute it to data acquisition and transformation on the LUS scanner side. To improve the transformation performance, a more powerful backend processor on the scanner side may be needed.

Due to different delays in streaming data from the two imaging devices, attention needs to be placed to data synchronization for AR visualization. One could synchronize the two data streams before performing the stereoscopic AR processing. If using this scheme, the system would have to delay video frames and the net latency would be 374 ms (sum of the three processing times in Fig. 4). The overall result would be a noticeable delay and visual disconnect between AR visualization and the real action related to the surgical procedure. Our system processes the two streaming data in a parallel manner (Fig. 4), i.e., the stereoscopic video is acquired and processed while acquiring the LUS data. In the final step of AR processing, the latest LUS image is overlaid on the prepared stereoscopic video and the video is rendered for 3D display. In this scheme, an 86-ms time lag results between the video and LUS imaging data but it is not noticeable. Our stereoscopic AR system thus uses the most up-to-date video and LUS images to produce real-time stereoscopic AR visualization.

The LUS image-to-video registration accuracy is critical from the standpoint of surgical safety. In our system, the primary determinant of accuracy is: how accurately the two imaging devices are calibrated. The stereo laparoscope calibration gave desirable result with a TRE of approximately 1 mm. It is intuitive to treat the stereo laparoscope as a stereo-camera system. However, this led to larger TRE than when treating it as two standalone cameras. The large TRE in the stereo-camera mode can be attributed to small separation between the left-eye and right-eye channel (1.04-mm IPD). Hence, a small error in camera calibration or localization of an image feature leads to a large TRE for the target point far from the reference frame. In our clinical applications, the desired LUS image-to-video registration accuracy is 2.5 mm. Future developments will attempt to further improve the accuracy.

The LUS calibration accuracy, TRE of approximately 1.5 mm, was acceptable using the current design. The long shaft of the LUS (Fig. 2) reduces calibration accuracy using optical tracking because, compared with traditional non-laparoscopic ultrasound probes, the LUS transducer is much farther from the reference frame affixed on its handle. Embedding an EM sensor close to the LUS transducer and replacing optical tracking with EM tracking may improve the accuracy of LUS calibration. No line-of-sight requirement of EM tracking is advantageous in the surgical setting as well.

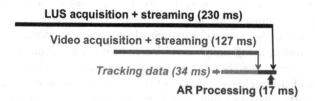

Fig. 4. The scheme for performing temporal synchronization.

In clinical practice, easy setup of the system in the OR is desirable to lower adoption barrier and to improve eventual success. The custom-designed fixtures can be easily snapped on to the two imaging devices by the current surgical team. These eliminated system recalibration as described. The rolling cart makes the system portable without the need for separately setting up the optical tracking system in the OR. These simplify the system setup and hence save expensive OR time.

5 Conclusion

Aiming to bring the stereoscopic AR technology into the clinic, we have developed a complete real-time stereoscopic AR visualization system for conventional laparoscopic surgery. Our ongoing work has addressed key issues of system latency, accuracy and portability. Our future work will include replacing optical tracking with EM tracking and further reducing the size and footprint of the system.

It is expected that the full development and clinical adoption of real-time stereoscopic AR visualization will make minimally invasive laparoscopic surgeries more precise and safer.

References

1. Leven, J., Burschka, D., Kumar, R., Zhang, G., Blumenkranz, S., Dai, X.D., Awad, M., Hager, G.D., Marohn, M., Choti, M., Hasser, C., Taylor, R.H.: DaVinci canvas: a telerobotic surgical system with integrated, robot-assisted, laparoscopic ultrasound capability. In: Duncan, J.S., Gerig, G. (eds.) MICCAI 2005. LNCS, vol. 3749, pp. 811–818. Springer, Heidelberg (2005)
2. Su, L.-M., Vagvolgyi, B.P., Agarwal, R., Reiley, C.E., Taylor, R.H., Hager, G.D.: Augmented reality during robot-assisted laparoscopic partial nephrectomy: toward real-time 3D-CT to stereoscopic video registration. Urology **73**(4), 896–900 (2009)
3. Cheung, C.L., Wedlake, C., Moore, J., Pautler, S.E., Ahmad, A., Peters, T.M.: Fusion of stereoscopic video and laparoscopic ultrasound for minimally invasive partial nephrectomy. Proc. SPIE **7261**, 726109–726110 (2009)
4. Cheung, C.L., Wedlake, C., Moore, J., Pautler, S.E., Peters, T.M.: Fused video and ultrasound images for minimally invasive partial nephrectomy: a phantom study. In: Jiang, T., Navab, N., Pluim, J.P., Viergever, M.A. (eds.) MICCAI 2010, Part III. LNCS, vol. 6363, pp. 408–415. Springer, Heidelberg (2010)
5. Teber, D., Guven, S., Simpfendörfer, T., Baumhauer, M., Güven, E.O., Yencilek, F., Gözen, A.S., Rassweiler, J.: Augmented reality: a new tool to improve surgical accuracy during laparoscopic partial nephrectomy? Preliminary in vitro and in vivo results. Eur. Urol. **56**(2), 332–338 (2009)
6. Simpfendörfer, T., Baumhauer, M., Müller, M., Gutt, C.N., Meinzer, H.P., Rassweiler, J.J., Guven, S., Teber, D.: Augmented reality visualization during laparoscopic radical prostatectomy. J. Endourol. **25**(12), 1841–1845 (2011)
7. Shekhar, R., Dandekar, O., Bhat, V., Philip, M., Lei, P., Godinez, C., Sutton, E., George, I., Kavic, S., Mezrich, R., Park, A.: Live augmented reality: a new visualization method for laparoscopic surgery using continuous volumetric computed tomography. Surg. Endosc. **24**(8), 1976–1985 (2010)

8. Zhang, Z.: A flexible new technique for camera calibration. IEEE Trans. Pattern Anal. Mach. Intell. **22**(11), 1330–1334 (2000)
9. Lasso, A., Heffter, T., Pinter, C., Ungi, T., Fichtinger, G.: Implementation of the PLUS open-source toolkit for translational research of ultrasound-guided intervention systems. In: MICCAI - Systems and Architectures for Computer Assisted Interventions, pp. 1–12 (2012)

Automatic Detection of Misalignment in Rigid 3D-2D Registration

Uroš Mitrović[(✉)], Žiga Špiclin, Boštjan Likar, and Franjo Pernuš

Faculty of Electrical Engineering, University of Ljubljana, Ljubljana, Slovenia
{uros.mitrovic, ziga.spiclin, bostjan.likar,
franjo.pernus}@fe.uni-lj.si

Abstract. Fusion of pre-interventional three-dimensional (3D) image to live two-dimensional (2D) image can facilitate minimally invasive image-guided interventions. For this purpose a number of 3D-2D registration methods related to different clinical contexts were proposed, however, their translation into clinical theater is still limited by lack of reliable and automatic detection of 3D-2D misalignment. In this paper, we presented a novel approach for verifying 3D-2D misalignment based on learned a priori knowledge using arbitrary similarity measure (SM) and single synthetic image (DRR). First, positions of local optima of SM using DRR image were found and characterized. On live 2D image, the local optima of SM were comparatively examined at the expected, previously learned positions. The approach was tested on publicly available image database of lumbar spine using state-of-the-art back-projection gradient-based SM. The results indicate that proposed approach successfully discriminated the "correct" from "poor" and "wrong" 3D-2D alignments in 100 % of cases.

Keywords: 3D-2D registration · Image guided surgery · Misalignment detection

1 Introduction

Minimally invasive, image-guided interventions (IGIs) are constantly replacing the invasive open surgery procedures and render the already minimally invasive procedures more accurate. Advantages of IGIs include shorter patient recovery times, greater patient comfort, lower risk of complications, and faster patient throughput. For diagnostic, intervention planning and simulation purposes a high quality three dimensional (3D) computed tomography (CT) or magnetic resonance (MR) image is typically acquired prior to the intervention. During the IGI, the interventional radiologist navigates his tools to the site of pathology relying only on one or at most two simultaneously acquired live two-dimensional (2D) fluoroscopic images. Due to overlapping of 3D structures and lack of depth information, navigation relying only on 2D images is a non-trivial task. An emerging solution is to exploit the positive aspects of 3D and 2D images by fusing the static 3D information with the temporal information of the live 2D fluoroscopic images [1]. The key step of data fusion is 3D-2D image registration.

M. Erdt et al. (Eds.): CLIP 2013, LNCS 8361, pp. 117–124, 2014.
DOI: 10.1007/978-3-319-05666-1_15, © Springer International Publishing Switzerland 2014

Over the last two decades, a large number of 3D-2D registration methods were proposed for different clinical contexts [2]. However, before introducing 3D-2D registration technology into clinical routine two key aspects must be fulfilled. First, the performance of 3D-2D registration method in terms of registration accuracy, robustness and computational complexity must meet clinical requirements. These should be validated on a large number of clinical image datasets. Second, a reliable method is required for automatically detecting misregistrations during IGI. For the validation of 3D-2D registration methods several publicly available image databases and protocols exist [3–5]. Even though that the automatic detection of image mis-alignment presents a crucial step for the translation of 3D-2D registration technology into clinical routine, it has not yet received much attention in the research community.

Crum et al. [6] estimated the image misalignment from the most significant voxel-scale present in scale-space residual image. Fedorov et al. [7] proposed a method for estimating registration error in mono-modal non-rigid image registration of MRI brain images using robust modification of Hausdorff distance measure. Möller and Posch [8] presented a hierarchical approach for automatic detection of registration error and underlying error sources based on robust analysis of difference image. Method for estimating translational errors for registration of binary 2D images is presented in [9]. Muenzing et al. [10] presented a supervised learning-based method for assessment of local image alignment at distinctive landmark points. The alignment was classified as "correct", "poor" or "wrong" based on a multi-feature classification scheme. An interesting approach for estimation of rigid-body registration quality using registration networks was proposed by Datteri and Dawant [11]. They demonstrated that regis-tration networks can identify registration error better than several popular similarity measures (SMs). In [12] the same authors extended their work for estimation of magnitude and location of error in non-rigid registration. The methods reviewed so far are limited to registration of images having the same dimensionality. Recently, Varnavas et al. [13] introduced a concept of virtual fiducial marker (VFM) and a gradient-difference based classification method for verifying the alignment quality in 3D-2D registration of images of vertebrae. Inserting the VFM requires the use of radio opaque ruler and acquisition of two additional 2D views which may present a limi-tation for some clinical contexts. On the other hand, estimation of alignment based on proposed gradient-difference based classification method seems to be suitable only for images of vertebrae and it is not immediately clear how to adopt the approach to other clinical contexts.

In this paper, we propose a new approach for assessment of 3D-2D registration alignment using a priori knowledge obtained from the pre-IGI 3D image and a single digitally reconstructed radiograph (DRR). The proposed approach is independent of the object of registration and of the selection of SM. The evaluation was performed using publicly available image database of spine phantom [3] and back-projection gradient-based (BGB) SM [14]. The results indicate that the proposed approach successfully discriminated between "correct", "poor" and "wrong" 3D-2D align-ments and achieved a 100 % rate of classification.

2 Method

The main idea of our approach is to estimate the behavior of 3D-2D registration SM on live 2D image (SM^{2D}) by observing the SM on DRR (SM^{DRR}). First, the positions of *distinctive* optima on SM^{DRR} and their relations to "gold standard" position are established, which we refer to as SM *mapping*. If the DRR and live 2D image depict the same anatomical structures in a similar way, then the distinctive optima on respective SM^{DRR} and SM^{2D} should have the same positions with respect to "gold standard" position. Finally, the quality of 3D-2D alignment is measured by similarity of SM^{DRR} and SM^{2D} at expected distinctive optima positions, referred to as SM *matching*. In the following, we describe SM mapping and matching.

SM Mapping. In this step, characteristic patterns on SM^{DRR} are found and their relations to the "gold standard" are established. By assuming coordinate system of 2D image as world coordinate system, the SM^{DRR} is then defined as function of six rigid body parameters $\mathbf{X} = (t_x, t_y, t_z, \omega_x, \omega_y, \omega_z)$ where t_x, t_y, ω_z represent in-plane parameters and t_z, ω_x, ω_y are out-of-plane parameters. According to [15] the SM^{DRR} is sampled on six-dimensional hypersphere of radius R_p and with center at "gold standard" position $\mathbf{X}_{GS}^{DRR}$ using NL_p sampling lines (Fig. 1 *left*). From the highest optimum per sampling line (besides "gold standard") Powell optimization method is ran and optimum *candidate* is obtained. Around each optimum candidate SM^{DRR} is then sampled on hypersphere of radius R using NL sampling lines and distinctiveness of optimum (DO) is calculated [15]. N_p optima with highest DOs and mutual distance greater than certain threshold R_{pp} are then selected as *distinctive* optima $\mathbf{X}_{Pi}^{DRR}$, $i = 1,2,...,N_p$. Finally, transformations $\mathbf{T}_{Pi}^{DRR}$, $i = 1,2,...,N_p$ which relate the "gold standard" position to the positions of distinctive optima are defined by $(\Delta t_x, \Delta t_y, \Delta t_z, \Delta \omega_x, \Delta \omega_y, \Delta \omega_z) = \mathbf{X}_{Pi}^{DRR} - \mathbf{X}_{GS}^{DRR}$. However, these transformations cannot be directly

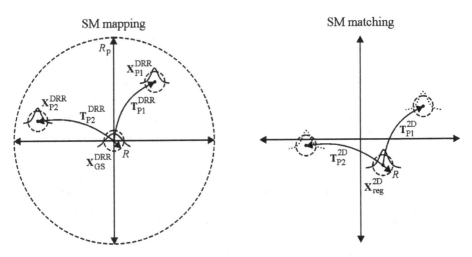

Fig. 1. Main steps of the proposed approach. Finding distinctive optima and associated transformations $\mathbf{T}_{Pi}^{DRR}$, $i=1,2,...,N_p$ on DRR image (*left*). Observing SM^{2D} at registered and positions defined by $\mathbf{T}_{Pi}^{2D}$ (*right*).

applied to real 2D image. Due to projective nature of 2D image, in-plane translations Δt_{xi} and Δt_{yi} are dependent on out-of-plane translation t_z (zoom). Knowing that 3D-2D registration methods in single view scenario are insensitive to zoom, Δt_{xi} and Δt_{yi} are typically under- or overestimated. By knowing zooms in "gold standard" and registered positions k_{GS} and k_{reg}, respectively, the Δt_{xi} and Δt_{yi} can be corrected as:

$$\Delta t'_{xi} = \frac{k_{GS}}{k_{reg}} \Delta t_{xi} \tag{1}$$

$$\Delta t'_{yi} = \frac{k_{GS}}{k_{reg}} \Delta t_{yi} \tag{2}$$

where $\Delta t'_{xi}$ and $\Delta t'_{yi}$ are corrected in-plane translations, which are used to calculate initial transformations $\mathbf{T}_{Pi}^{2D'}$, $i = 1,2,...,N_p$. As optima on SM^{2D} are not necessarily at exact position defined by $\mathbf{T}_{Pi}^{2D'}$, Powell method is used to find closest distinctive optimum. Finally, if the distance between optimized position and initial position is smaller than some threshold R_{opt}, the optimized position is used to define final transformation $\mathbf{T}_{Pi}^{2D}$, otherwise $\mathbf{T}_{Pi}^{2D} = \mathbf{T}_{Pi}^{2D'}$.

SM Matching. Based on SM mapping, SM^{2D} is sampled on registered position $\mathbf{X}_{reg}^{2D}$ and positions defined by $\mathbf{T}_{Pi}^{2D}$, using the same sampling points as for SM^{DRR} (Fig. 1 *right*). If the registered position $\mathbf{X}_{reg}^{2D}$ is close to the "gold standard", the distinctive optima on SM^{2D} will be at positions defined by $\mathbf{T}_{Pi}^{2D}$ and thus difference between SM^{DRR} and SM^{2D} will be small. Similarly, for larger registration errors $\mathbf{T}_{Pi}^{2D}$ will point to random behavior of SM^{2D} and thus the difference will be higher (Fig. 2). To quantify the degree of 3D-2D alignment we employ two measures. First, is the average absolute difference between SM^{DRR} and SM^{2D} at N_p+1 optima positions defined as:

$$\Delta SM = \frac{1}{N_p + 1} \sum_{i=1}^{Np+1} \left| SM_{pi}^{DRR} - SM_{pi}^{2D} \right| \tag{3}$$

where SM_{Pi}^{DRR} and SM_{Pi}^{2D} are values of SM at i-th optimum position using either DRR or 2D image, respectively. Second, is average value of DO calculated at registered and positions defined by $\mathbf{T}_{Pi}^{2D}$ referred to as DO_{avg}. Note, that according to [15] the values of SM_{Pi}^{DRR} and SM_{Pi}^{2D} used for calculation of ΔSM and DO_{avg} are normalized to $[0, 1]$ interval.

Parameter Values. The values of $NL_p = 50$ and $R_p = 30$ mm were used to sample SM^{DRR} in the SM mapping step. Each optima was sampled with $NL = 25$ lines on $R = 5$ mm hypersphere. Distance between two sample points in all our calculations was set to 0.2 mm. Minimal mutual distance between two optima R_{pp} was set to 5 mm of mean reprojection distance (mRPD). The maximal allowed distance between initial and optimized position R_{opt} was set to 2 mm of mRPD.

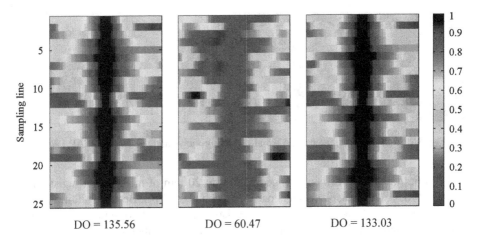

$$\text{DO} = 135.56 \qquad \text{DO} = 60.47 \qquad \text{DO} = 133.03$$

Fig. 2. *From left to right:* SM^{2D} for "correct", "wrong" registration and SM^{DRR} of the same distinctive optima. Associated DO values are given below.

3   Experiments and Results

The BGB 3D-2D registration method proposed by Tomaževič et al. [14] was used to demonstrate proof of our proposed concept. It was applied to the 3D and two 2D images of cadaveric lumbar spine using single 2D image a time [3]. In the following, the BGB method, evaluation database, evaluation methodology and the results of the proposed approach are presented.

Gradient-Based Back-Projection Method (BGB). The BGB method is based on matching 3D gradient vectors representing surface normals and back-projected gradient vectors defined in 2D image by the position of the X-ray source and current position of 3D surface normals. In the pre-processing step, the 3D volume and 2D image were blurred with a Gaussian filter and the resulting 3D image was isotropically resampled. For calculation of volume gradients, the 3D Canny edge detector was applied, while the 2D gradients were calculated using a simple central-differences kernel. For each 3D gradient, its corresponding back-projected 2D gradient was defined and their magnitudes and angles were used to calculate the similarity measure. The six parameters, defining the optimal rigid transformation between the volume gradients and the back-projected 2D gradients, were searched for by optimizing the SM with the Powell's method.

Evaluation Database and Methodology. For testing of our approach, CT and two X-ray images acquired at approximately lateral (LAT) and anterior-posterior (AP) views from publicly available cadaveric lumbar spine image database were used [3] (Fig. 3). The CT image, was divided into five sub volumes comprising only single L1-L5 vertebra.

Each sub volume was 100 time randomly displaced from the "gold standard" position in the range of $[-20, 20]$ mm and $[-10, 10]$ degrees, respectively. This

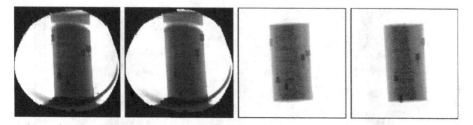

Fig. 3. *From left to right:* the LAT and AP X-ray views and the LAT and AP DRR.

resulted in initial displacements ranged from 0 to 20 mm of mean target registration error (mTRE), with 5 displacements per 1 mm subinterval [4]. Besides, additional six initial displacements were generated by registering each sub volume to non-corresponding vertebra on 2D image, which represent the most difficult 3D-2D registration cases. The sub volumes were registered to a single 2D image a time, resulting in 1060 registrations in total. The registrations were divided into three classes "correct", "poor" and "wrong" depending on mRPD. mRPD below 1 mm denotes to "correct", mRPD between 1 and 2 mm denotes to "poor", while mRPD above 2 mm denotes to "wrong" registration. The classification performance was measured by area under the receiver operator characteristic (ROC) curve.

Results. The results were obtained using $N_p = 5$ distinctive optima (besides "gold standard"), with BGB SM^{DRR} mapped on DRRs generated using "gold standard" position of pre-IGI CT image (Fig. 3). The scatter plots and classification performances using ΔSM and DO_{avg} are given in Fig. 4 and Table 1, respectively. Besides, results using value of SM^{2D} and DO solely at registered position are also given in the same figure and table.

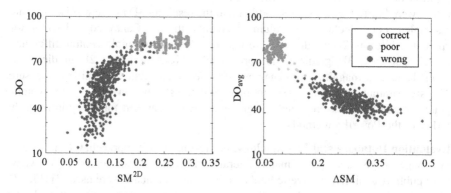

Fig. 4. Scatter plots of registration results using solely registered position (*left*) and with proposed approach (*right*).

Table 1. Area under ROC curve of ΔSM, DO_{avg}, SM^{2D} and DO for classification "correct" vs. "poor" and "correct" vs. "wrong" registration.

	ΔSM	DO_{avg}	SM^{2D}	DO
"correct" vs. "poor"	97.04	**100**	62.94	82.10
"correct" vs. "wrong"	**100**	**100**	99.49	99.76

4 Discussion and Conclusion

A large number of 3D-2D registration methods were proposed for the purposes of application in IGI. Usually, the performance of these methods was evaluated against "gold standard" registration, and then their accuracy and capture range were determined by generating random displacements from the "gold standard" position. However, in reality, pre-IGI 3D image can be displaced significantly out of range of 3D-2D registration method, which can thus get easily trapped in local optima. Therefore, a reliable automatic verification of the registration alignment is required, before introducing the 3D-2D registration technology into clinical theater.

In the proposed automatic registration verification approach, we exploited the information about the position of local optima and the behavior of SM about the local optima yielding a locally characterized SM. This was carried out by generating a single DRR from a pre-IGI 3D image and establishing relations between the positions of local optima and the "gold standard" position. Moreover, as the DRR image should resemble the live 2D image, similar behavior of SM is expected on both images about the positions of local optima and their relation to the "gold standard" position. To prove our concept we employed state-of-the-art BGB 3D-2D registration method and applied it to publicly available image database of cadaveric lumbar spine phantom. The CT images of L1-L5 vertebra were registered to two live 2D images using single 2D image a time. In total 1060 registrations were performed and divided into three classes: "correct", "poor" and "wrong". Obtained results showed that using solely the value of SM is not sufficient to discriminate between "correct" and "wrong" registrations. On the other hand, the measures based on a priori knowledge, ΔSM and DO_{avg} successfully discriminated "correct" from "wrong" registration in 100 % of cases (Table 1). Besides, DO_{avg} seemed to be more sensitive to the misalignment as it also successfully discriminated "correct" from "poor" registrations in 100 % of cases.

The performance of the proposed approach depends mainly on similarity between DRR and live 2D image, and knowledge about the zoom of 3D object in "gold standard", which can usually be acquired from the DICOM header. The DRR and live 2D image should depict those anatomical structures and features, which will guide the registration in a comparable way, and furthermore that both 2D images are acquired with a comparable pose of the pre-IGI 3D image. The advantage of the proposed approach is that transformations T_{Pi}^{DRR} are inherently invariant on selection of translations t_x, t_y, t_z and in-plane rotation ω_z of pre-IGI 3D image used for generating the DRR. However, the proposed approach is sensitive to the error in the out-of-plane rotations ω_x, ω_y which we will carefully examine in our future work. Finally, the proposed approach can be used with arbitrary SM and object of registration, therefore, we plan to investigate its performance using different SMs and different image databases.

Acknowledgments. This research was supported by the Ministry of Education, Science, Culture and Sport, Republic of Slovenia, under grants L2-2023, L2-9758, J2-0716, J2-2246, and P2-0232.

References

1. Copeland, A.D., Mangoubi, R.S., Desai, M.N., Mitter, S.K., Malek, A.M.: Spatio-temporal data fusion for 3D+T image reconstruction in cerebral angiography. IEEE Trans. Med. Imaging **29**, 1238–1251 (2010)
2. Markelj, P., Tomaževič, D., Likar, B., Pernuš, F.: A review of 3D/2D registration methods for image-guided interventions. Med. Image Anal. **16**, 642–661 (2012)
3. Tomaževič, D., Likar, B., Pernuš, F.: "Gold standard" data for evaluation and comparison of 3D/2D registration methods. Comput. Aided Surg. **9**, 137–144 (2004)
4. Van de Kraats, E., Penney, G., Tomaževič, D., van Walsum, T., Niessen, W.: Standardized evaluation methodology for 2-D-3-D registration. IEEE Trans. Med. Imaging **24**, 1177–1189 (2005)
5. Mitrović, U., Špiclin, Ž., Likar, B., Pernuš, F.: 3D-2D registration of cerebral angiograms: a method and evaluation on clinical images. IEEE Trans. Med. Imaging **32**, 1550–1563 (2013). (Early Access Online)
6. Crum, W.R., Griffin, L.D., Hawkes, D.J.: Automatic estimation of error in voxel-based registration. In: Barillot, C., Haynor, D.R., Hellier, P. (eds.) MICCAI 2004. LNCS, vol. 3216, pp. 821–828. Springer, Heidelberg (2004)
7. Fedorov, A., Billet, E., Prastawa, M., Gerig, G., Radmanesh, A., Warfield, S.K., Kikinis, R., Chrisochoides, N.: Evaluation of brain MRI alignment with the robust Hausdorff distance measures. In: Bebis, G., Boyle, R., Parvin, B., Koracin, D., Remagnino, P., Porikli, F., Peters, J., Klosowski, J., Arns, L., Chun, Y.K., Rhyne, T.-M., Monroe, L. (eds.) Advances in Visual Computing, pp. 594–603. Springer, Heidelberg (2008)
8. Möller, B., Posch, S.: An integrated analysis concept for errors in image registration. Pattern Recognit. Image Anal. **18**, 201–206 (2008)
9. Simonson, K.M., Drescher, S.M., Tanner, F.R.: A statistics-based approach to binary image registration with uncertainty analysis. IEEE Trans. Pattern Anal. Mach. Intell. **29**, 112–125 (2007)
10. Muenzing, S.E.A., van Ginneken, B., Murphy, K., Pluim, J.P.W.: Supervised quality assessment of medical image registration: application to intra-patient CT lung registration. Med. Image Anal. **16**, 1521–1531 (2012)
11. Datteri, R., Dawant, B.M.: Estimation of rigid-body registration quality using registration networks. Proc. SPIE **8314**, 831419 (2012)
12. Datteri, R.D., Dawant, B.M.: Automatic detection of the magnitude and spatial location of error in non-rigid registration. In: Dawant, B.M., Christensen, G.E., Fitzpatrick, J.M., Rueckert, D. (eds.) Biomedical Image Registration, pp. 21–30. Springer, Heidelberg (2012)
13. Varnavas, A., Carrell, T., Penney, G.: Increasing the automation of a 2D-3D registration system. IEEE Trans. Med. Imaging **32**, 387–399 (2013)
14. Tomaževič, D., Likar, B., Slivnik, T., Pernuš, F.: 3-D/2-D registration of CT and MR to X-ray images. IEEE Trans. Med. Imaging **22**, 1407–1416 (2003)
15. Škerl, D., Likar, B., Pernuš, F.: A protocol for evaluation of similarity measures for rigid registration. IEEE Trans. Med. Imaging **25**, 779–791 (2006)

Prototype Design and Phantom Evaluation of a Device for Co-registered MRI/TRUS Imaging of the Prostate

Andriy Fedorov[1]([✉]), Sang-Eun Song[1], Tina Kapur[1], Robert Owen[2],
Emily Neubauer Sugar[3], Paul Nguyen[3], William M. Wells III[1],
and Clare M. Tempany[1]

[1] Department of Radiology, Brigham and Women's Hospital,
Harvard Medical School, Boston, MA 02115, USA
`fedorov@bwh.harvard.edu`
[2] BK Medical, Peabody, MA 01960, USA
[3] Department of Radiation Oncology, Brigham and Women's Hospital,
Harvard Medical School, Boston, MA 02115, USA

Abstract. Magnetic Resonance Imaging (MRI) and transrectal Ultrasound (TRUS) are both used in imaging interventions in men suspected of having and with prostate cancer for diagnosis as well as treatment. Due to the widespread availability and ease of use of TRUS, it is widely acknowledged that availability of spatially registered MRI/TRUS data could provide the optimal combination for characterization of prostate tissue and interventional guidance. To provide such spatially aligned data, we propose a device to support co-registered acquisition of MRI and TRUS data while maintaining a stable configuration (shape) of the prostate. We present the design and evaluation of a custom sleeve that can be introduced transrectally, and can accommodate both TRUS and endorectal MRI probes. Our experiments on a phantom have demonstrated that imaging with this sleeve did not compromise differentiation of internal structures and did not affect the quality of the MR acquisition. Reduction of the signal and contrast were however observed and quantified in the TRUS data. Further evaluation and modification of the device necessary for possible patient studies are discussed.

Keywords: Prostate cancer · Image-guided interventions · Magnetic resonance imaging · Transrectal ultrasound · Image registration · Tissue characterization · Phantom evaluation

1   Introduction

Prostate cancer (PCa) is the most common non-cutaneous malignancy in men in the USA [1]. Imaging has a unique role in the clinical management of this disease. Transrectal ultrasound (TRUS) is the most commonly used method for image guided biopsy of the prostate gland; it is widely used for collection of core biopsy

M. Erdt et al. (Eds.): CLIP 2013, LNCS 8361, pp. 125–133, 2014.
DOI: 10.1007/978-3-319-05666-1_16, © Springer International Publishing Switzerland 2014

samples in sextant approaches, and for guiding treatment procedures. The use of TRUS has expanded beyond routine clinical B-mode acquisitions to guide treatment, to research in US elastography and analysis of radiofrequency (RF) signal for tissue characterization [2]. Meanwhile, Magnetic Resonance Imaging (MRI) is most commonly used for detection, localization and staging of PCa [3, 4]. The complementary utility of these two imaging approaches is recognized and has motivated the development of systems that augment intra-procedural TRUS for real-time imaging of the gland with pre-procedural MRI clearly showing the confirmed or suspected cancer regions. In practice, development of such systems is challenging due to lack of spatial alignment between the MR and US modalities. To alleviate this problem, we report our initial experience in the development of a device to reduce deformation of the prostate by providing a fixed physical setup during the acquisition of MRI and TRUS data.

One of the challenges in supporting joint MRI/US visualization is the difference in the spatial configuration, i.e. shape, of the prostate between the TRUS and MRI imaging sessions. Each imaging modality is associated with its own unique deformation of the gland tissues. As a result, some form of registration between the MRI and TRUS imaging is typically required to provide meaningful joint visualization. Due to the significant differences between the MRI and TRUS images, practical registration approaches are often augmented by the use of various forms of tracking and segmentation of the prostate gland to simplify the registration problem. Early approaches to MRI/TRUS registration were based on rigid alignment using anatomical landmarks [5]. More commonly, the registration is based on aligning boundaries of the prostate segmented in MRI and TRUS. Several surface-based registration approaches have been proposed [6,7]. Hu et al. developed a model-to-image registration method that relies on biomechanical simulation to estimate the most likely deformation in the planning stage of the procedure [8]. Over the last years, several systems have become available commercially to support MRI/TRUS image fusion [9]. Most of these commercial systems rely on the segmentation of the prostate gland to provide non-rigid deformation between MRI and TRUS. While there is strong evidence that MRI/TRUS fusion improves accuracy of biopsy guidance for PCa detection, the targeting accuracy of the fusion systems is difficult to assess. Commonly used error quantification approaches only utilize manually identified corresponding features that are consistent in MRI and TRUS. Due to the differences between the MR and US modalities, localization of the corresponding features is challenging and time-consuming, limiting the applicability of the approach.

In this article we propose an alternative to commonly used registration of images obtained from MRI and TRUS. Our method relies on a custom device that can maintain the spatial arrangement of the prostate between the MRI and TRUS imaging sessions. As an expected result, deformable registration of the two imaging modalities can be eliminated, thus, a rigid coordinate system transformation between the two images collected by the respective modalities should be sufficient for spatial alignment. Such a device can facilitate intra-procedural tracking of the target, providing valuable data for joint characterization of the MRI/TRUS and for validation of image-based deformable registration.

The goals of this paper are twofold. First, we present the technical considerations and the initial design of a device to maintain consistent spatial arrangement of the prostate gland. Second, we report a phantom study that we performed, using this device, to establish the feasibility of MRI and TRUS imaging, and to evaluate the quality of the collected images.

2   Methods

Our initial design of the Adjustable Sleeve Template Assembly (ASTA) device was conceived to support consistent spatial arrangement of the prostate and interchangeable MRI/TRUS imaging during two targeted transperineal interventions – template-based biopsy, and implantation of low-dose radioactive seeds in prostate brachytherapy. To achieve this goal, the complete ASTA device would include (1) a sleeve, constructed to be MR safe and US-transparent, to interchangeably accommodate both the MRI endorectal coil and the TRUS probe, (2) the biopsy/brachytherapy grid template rigidly attached to the sleeve, and (3) a calibration device, such as Z-frame [10]. Consistent position of the ASTA would be maintained by semi-rigid mechanical coupling to the procedure table. In this article, we focus on the development of the sleeve component of ASTA, and evaluation of the image quality when such a sleeve is used.

Design of the ASTA Sleeve. Our design was intended to accommodate two imaging probes interchangeably: a rigid transrectal MR coil (Hologic Endo MRI Coil, Hologic Inc, Bedford, MA), measuring 25 mm at its widest cross-section, and a transrectal ultrasound probe (BK 8848, BK Medical, Peabody, MA) measuring 20 mm at its widest cross-section. A sleeve was fabricated from polymethylpentene (TPX), a material with acoustic impedance similar to tissue [11]. Sleeve thickness was set to 1.8 mm, resulting in sleeve outer diameter of 29 mm (25.4 mm inside diameter to accommodate the coil). To account for the differences in the outer diameter between the MR coil and US transducer, a saline-filled endocavity balloon (Civco Medical Solutions, Kalona, IA) was used during TRUS imaging through the sleeve. As an FDA-approved clinical device, the endocavity balloon serves a dual purpose: it improves acoustic coupling between the tissue and the transducer surface, and, when necessary, pushes the prostate gland to match the coverage field of the brachytherapy template. In our scenario, the balloon was used to ensure acoustic coupling between the transducer and the sleeve. The components involved in the experimental setup are shown in Fig. 1.

Image Acquisition. Ultrasound imaging Our experiments for evaluating the feasibility imaging, and the quality of resulting images, utilized a standard multi-modality prostate phantom (model 053-MM, CIRS, Norfolk, VA). The phantom is constructed with different types of materials to emulate imaging contrast between anatomical structures, including the prostate gland, urethra and lesions. TRUS imaging was performed using the BK ProFocus system and the transverse array of

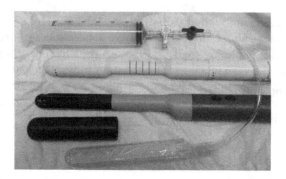

Fig. 1. Components used in the experimental setup. From top to bottom shown are (1) a syringe connected with the endocavity balloon (Civco); (2) rigid transrectal MRI coil (Hologic); (3) transrectal ultrasound probe (BK Medical); (4) custom fabricated TPX sleeve.

the 8848 transrectal probe with the endocavity balloon mounted according to the manufacturer instructions. The experiments were performed with and without the sleeve to compare image quality. Each of the experiments was repeated 10 times, with the transducer reinserted during each experiment to evaluate the repeatability of the measurements. Ultrasound gel (Aquasonic, Parker Labs, Farfield, NJ) was used to enhance acoustic coupling of the surfaces. Identical acquisition settings were used for the imaging experiments with and without the sleeve (gain 80 %, dynamic range 79 dB, frequency 12 MHz, depth 5.4 cm, identical range and depth of the focal interval). Image collection was facilitated by the open source Public Library for UltraSound research (PLUS)[1] [12].

MR Imaging. MR imaging experiments were conducted in a 3 Tesla scanner (Siemens Magnetom Verio, Erlangen, Germany). Imaging was performed using the commercially available tabletop attachment (Hologic Inc, Bedford, MA) to the scanner table. Two pelvic array coils were placed above and below the phantom, and the rigid endorectal coil was placed in the phantom rectum. Imaging was performed using multi-slice Turbo Spin Echo T2-weighted sequence (TR/TE = 2700 ms/106 ms; acquisition matrix = 280×280; flip angle = 48°; field of view = 200×200 mm^2; slice thickness = 3 mm; receiver bandwidth = 252 Hz/pixel; imaging time: 1 min). MR imaging was repeated 5 times both with and without ASTA sleeve, with the endorectal coil reinserted for each imaging session.

Image Quality Assessment. Images of the phantom corresponding to approximately the same transverse plane were assessed. A consistent transverse location was selected such that the slice covered the widest cross-section of the specific lesion implanted in the phantom. To quantitatively measure the degradation in image quality caused by the ASTA sleeve, we used two measures:

1. Average signal value in the regions of interest (TRUS only). For US images, signal intensity relates to the energy of the returning ultrasound waves. There-

---

[1] Public Library for UltraSound research (PLUS), http://plustoolkit.org.

fore, reduction in grayscale values is a measure of signal loss due to the introduction of extra layers between the scanned object and transducer surface.

2. Pairwise contrast to noise (CNR) measure:

$$CNR = \frac{2(\mu_1 - \mu_2)^2}{(\sigma_1^2 + \sigma_2^2)}, \tag{1}$$

where μ_1 and μ_2 are the mean intensity values, and σ_1 and σ_2 are standard deviation values for the two regions. CNR was measured pairwise between the prostate, urethra and lesion in the phantom.

3   Results

Using visual examination of the acquired images, we confirmed that MRI and TRUS imaging through the ASTA sleeve was feasible. Acoustic coupling during US imaging was established in all experiments and no gross artifacts were observed. Image contrast was sufficient to differentiate all the phantom structures considered in the evaluation (prostate, urethra and lesions regions). Representative images are shown in Fig. 2. US images collected through the balloon/sleeve assembly had noticeably reduced signal, were noisier and had reduced sharpness of the boundary between the distinctive phantom structures, based on visual inspection, as can be observed in Fig. 2 (top row). A bright double halo surrounding the region corresponding to the probe location was apparent in the MR images, however no noticeable degradation of the MR image quality was observed by introducing the sleeve.

The results of the quantitative assessment of the collected data are summarized in Fig. 3 and Table 1. Measurements of the signal strength agreed with

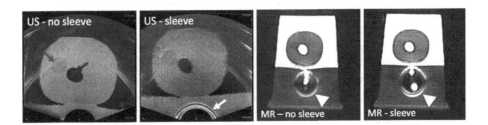

Fig. 2. Representative US and MR images of the multimodality prostate phantom. The slice shown corresponds to approximately the same transverse position relative to the phantom geometry. CNR measurements were performed pairwise between the lesion (red arrow), urethra (green arrow) and prostate regions (structure enclosing lesion and urethra). Strong reflection artifact near the surface of the TRUS probe (white arrow) corresponds to the saline-filled endocavity balloon, TPX sleeve and the layers of gel that were used to ensure acoustic coupling between the surfaces. Single and double bright circles observed in MRI (white arrowhead) are due to the signal from the acoustic gel surrounding the coil and the sleeve (Color figure online).

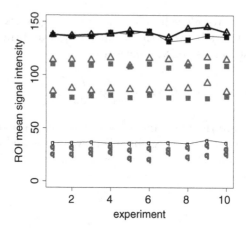

Fig. 3. Average signal measured from the regions of interest defined in lesion (square marker), prostate (triangle) and urethra (circle) areas. Colors correspond to the images acquires using transducer without introducing any additional layers (black), using endocavity balloon alone (blue), and together with the TPX sleeve (red). Reduction of signal introduced by addition of extra layers is apparent (Color figure online).

Table 1. Quantitative assessment of the US and MR image contrast between the lesion (region 1), urethra (2) and prostate (3) phantom tissue types. Mean and standard deviation reported for the pairwise combinations of the considered regions.

Modality	Summary statistics	CNR, no sleeve			CNR, sleeve		
		1–2	1–3	2–3	1–2	1–3	2–3
US	mean	144	0.2	182	47	0.5	71
US	STD	29	0.4	40	9	0.3	10
MR	mean	952	0.7	1004	804	1.8	826
MR	STD	397	0.5	420	215	2.8	217

the visual assessment of US images, as we observed reduction of the signal that was reproducible across the experiments. Averaged over 10 experiments, the mean grayscale values measured in the TRUS images were (for the three regions of interest considered) 136, 37 and 139 when the transducer was used without extra attachments, 109, 25 and 114 units when endocavity balloon was used, and 75, 36 and 87 units when we added the TPX sleeve. Differences between the signal values for the MR images were minimal. CNR measurements showed reduction of CNR when balloon/TPX sleeve were introduced.

4   Discussion and Conclusions

In this study we introduced a prototype of a simple sleeve-based device to facilitate co-registered acquisition of endorectal MRI/TRUS imaging of the prostate. The motivation for this device is to maintain the prostate in a consistent position and shape so that there is minimal or no effect on the prostate configuration due to removal or introduction of imaging probes. Our study focused on the preliminary evaluation of technical feasibility of the prototype and assessment of the image quality. We confirmed experimentally that imaging of the phantom with the sleeve assembly was feasible using both MR and US, does not introduce severe artifacts, and does not compromise the ability of the operator to differentiate the structures of interest in the phantom. This was confirmed even for the lesion structure of the phantom, which has rather low contrast relative to its surrounding.

Our experimental evaluation also showed that introduction of the extra layers, even when those layers are fabricated from materials with acoustic properties similar to tissue, resulted in reduction of signal strength and contrast in the US images. Such signal loss is not only due to the presence of the extra TPX/saline layers, but also due to the intermediate layers of gel used for acoustic coupling. There are several observations related to this reduction of signal and image contrast. First, we note that the loss of signal strength due to the presence of a TPX sleeve appears to be comparable with that caused by the saline-filled endocavity balloon (as can be seen in Fig. 3), an FDA-approved product for our clinical scenario. This leads us to conjecture that the signal loss we are introducing with the TPX is comparable to what is considered acceptable clinically. Second, we used identical setup and image acquisition parameters for the experiments with and without the sleeve. An increase in the TRUS gain settings in the experiments that used the sleeve can potentially improve CNR. Finally, we note that while the phantom experiments reported in this study allow us to understand and quantify some of the technical issues related to image acquisition, further investigations are needed in order to understand the applicability of the device in the patient studies.

There are several specific clinical usage scenarios where a sleeve-based device such as the one presented can be used. For example, an MRI scan with the device in place can be obtained at the beginning of a procedure, followed by an US scan. After that the device can be removed, and targets identified in MRI can be tracked by registration between the initial, possibly 3D reconstructed, US, with the intra-procedural US data. Alternatively, volumetric TRUS study can be performed immediately after the MRI scan at the time of the diagnostic exam, in advance of the intervention. As a second example, RF TRUS data that is acquired in near-perfect alignment with mpMRI can be used for characterization of the prostate tissue. To implement such scenarios, further engineering efforts are underway. For instance, ASTA design must be able to maintain the sleeve at a fixed position while imaging probes are exchanged. A multi-modality operating room, such as AMIGO at BWH[2], would be ideal for evaluation of the setup, as the patient lithotomy position needs to be maintained while the patient is moved out of the scanner bore.

---

[2] The Advanced Multimodality Image-Guided Operating (AMIGO) Suite, Brigham and Women's Hospital, Boston, USA, http://www.ncigt.org/pages/AMIGO.

The design evaluated in this study represents only one of the prototypes we have considered. Alternative designs that do not introduce extra layers between the ultrasound transducer and the tissue have been tested and will be included in future evaluations. The US imaging experiments were performed utilizing only the transverse array of the probe. Additional experiments may be performed to evaluate the feasibility of the sagittal array scanning and the quality of the 3D reconstructed TRUS volumes.

In conclusion, we have presented initial results in developing and evaluating a device for co-registered MR/TRUS prostate imaging. The images of the phantom obtained while using the sleeve have reasonable quality. Further evaluation and modification of the device are planned prior to clinical use. ASTA can provide MR/US data with minimal misalignment and it can be valuable for improved understanding of prostate tissue characterization, development of joint MR/US appearance models of prostate, and improved accuracy of image-guided prostate interventions.

Acknowledgments. This work was supported in part by NIH grants R01 CA111288 and P41 EB015898. We thank Iris Elliott for her contribution to the discussions related to the use of MR coil.

References

1. American Cancer Society: Cancer Facts & Figures (2013)
2. Moradi, M., Mousavi, P., Abolmaesumi, P.: Computer-aided diagnosis of prostate cancer with emphasis on ultrasound-based approaches: a review. Ultrasound Med. Biol. **33**(7), 1010–1028 (2007)
3. Turkbey, B., et al.: Multiparametric 3T prostate magnetic resonance imaging to detect cancer: histopathological correlation using prostatectomy specimens processed in customized magnetic resonance imaging based molds. J. Urol. **186**(5), 1818–1824 (2011)
4. Langer, D.L., van der Kwast, T.H., Evans, A.J., Trachtenberg, J., Wilson, B.C., Haider, M.A.: Prostate cancer detection with multi-parametric MRI: logistic regression analysis of quantitative T2, diffusion-weighted imaging, and dynamic contrast-enhanced MRI. J. Magn. Reson. Imaging : JMRI **30**(2), 327–334 (2009)
5. Kaplan, I., Oldenburg, N.E., Meskell, P., Blake, M., Church, P., Holupka, E.J.: Real time MRI-ultrasound image guided stereotactic prostate biopsy. Magn. Reson. Imaging **20**(3), 295–299 (2002)
6. Daanen, V., Gastaldo, J., Giraud, J.Y., Fourneret, P., Descotes, J.L., Bolla, M., Collomb, D., Troccaz, J.: MRI/TRUS data fusion for brachytherapy. Int. J. Med. Robot. + Comput. Assist. Surg. MRCAS **2**(3), 256–261 (2006)
7. Narayanan, R., Kurhanewicz, J., Shinohara, K., Crawford, E.D., Simoneau, A., Suri, J.S.: MRI-ultrasound registration for targeted prostate biopsy. In: 2009 IEEE International Symposium on Biomedical Imaging: From Nano to Macro, Boston, Massachusetts, USA, pp. 991–994. IEEE Press (June 2009)
8. Hu, Y., Ahmed, H.U., Taylor, Z., Allen, C., Emberton, M., Hawkes, D., Barratt, D.: MR to ultrasound registration for image-guided prostate interventions. Med. Image Anal. **16**(3), 687–703 (2012)

 9. Marks, L., Young, S., Natarajan, S.: MRI-ultrasound fusion for guidance of targeted prostate biopsy. Curr. Opin. Urol. **23**(1), 43–50 (2013)
10. DiMaio, Simon P., Samset, Eigil, Fischer, G., Iordachita, Iulian I., Fichtinger, Gabor, Jolesz, Ferenc A., Tempany, Clare M.C.: Dynamic MRI scan plane control for passive tracking of instruments and devices. In: Ayache, Nicholas, Ourselin, Sébastien, Maeder, Anthony (eds.) MICCAI 2007, Part II. LNCS, vol. 4792, pp. 50–58. Springer, Heidelberg (2007)
11. Madsen, E.L., Deaner, M.E., Mehi, J.: Properties of phantom tissuelike polymethylpentene in the frequency range 20–70 MHZ. Ultrasound Med. Biol. **37**(8), 1327–1339 (2011)
12. Lasso, A., Heffter, T., Pinter, C., Ungi, T., Fichtinger, G.: Implementation of the PLUS open-source toolkit for translational research of ultrasound-guided intervention systems. In: The MIDAS Journal – Systems and Architectures for Computer-Assisted Interventions Workshop, MICCAI 2012, pp. 1–12 (2012)

Modelling Smooth Intensity Changes in the Putamen for Diagnosis of Sporadic Creutzfeldt-Jakob Disease

S. Bouyagoub[1(✉)], I.C. Cimpan[2], S.A. Hojjatoleslami[2], A. Kume[2], Y.H. Mah[1], and A.C.F. Colchester[1,2]

[1] East Kent Hospitals University Foundation Trust, Canterbury, UK
[2] University of Kent, Canterbury, UK
samira.bouyagoub@nhs.net,
a.colchester@kent.ac.uk

Abstract. The putamen, one of the deep grey matter structures in the brain, is unusual in that MRI intensities vary smoothly within the structure. We develop a geometric and intensity model of the putamen, and in averaged images from 60 CJD patients and non-CJD clinical controls we show these smooth changes clearly. In the axial plane, there is a linear decrease of T2 intensity from anterior to posterior in the central part of the putamen. The gradient is significantly higher in sporadic CJD, but not in variant CJD, than controls. We show that gradient quantification would give good sensitivity and specificity, making this suitable as a simple screening test for sporadic CJD. However, the data are preliminary; a wider database of patients and further statistical analyses are needed for a robust definition of the clinical role of the test.

Keywords: Putamen · Gradient · MRI · Sporadic CJD diagnosis · Variant CJD

1 Introduction

Creutzfeldt-Jakob disease (CJD) is a rare fatal neurological disease in which an abnormal prion protein accumulates in the brain. The commonest form occurs worldwide, with no identifiable environmental or genetic explanation, and is referred to as sporadic CJD (sCJD). However, CJD can also be transmitted like an infection from one individual to another, and transmission of the related disease of cattle (BSE) to man is known to have occurred to cause variant CJD (vCJD). CJD usually presents with cognitive deficits that can mimic common forms of dementia and clinical suspicion of the diagnosis can be delayed. By the time of diagnosis, extensive infective tissue has accumulated in the individual, and to enable precautionary measures to be taken to reduce risk of transmission through contact with infective tissue, there is a strong public health requirement to improve early diagnosis with non-invasive tests.

MRI is an important diagnostic tool in suspected cases. In vCJD, increased signal intensity in the posterior thalamus (the pulvinar sign) is seen in a high proportion of cases and is both sensitive and specific. In sCJD, high signal occurs in the cortex,

M. Erdt et al. (Eds.): CLIP 2013, LNCS 8361, pp. 134–142, 2014.
DOI: 10.1007/978-3-319-05666-1_17, © Springer International Publishing Switzerland 2014

caudate nucleus and putamen more than in the thalamus, but the findings vary considerably in different cases [1]. Most publications describe visual appearances (e.g. [2]); very few have explored the potential of intensity quantification [3, 4]. An important study of a small number of sCJD and vCJD patients segmented the deep nuclei by co-registration with an atlas and evaluated different approaches to intensity normalisation and detection of intensity abnormalities, with good results [5]. A limitation of this study was the use of normal subjects as controls, whereas in a clinical context the question is whether patients with CJD can be distinguished from those with a similar initial presentation (such as a rapidly progressive dementia) but who do not have CJD. Another study reported a gradient of intensity change within the putamen in sCJD patients, which was estimated by averaging intensities in the anterior putamen and comparing this with the more posterior part; this had good performance against non-CJD dementia controls [6]. Despite the promise of improving diagnostic accuracy, quantitative MRI methods so far have not been adopted in clinical practice.

The challenges for quantification include the substantial variability of MRI intensities between different scanners, the lack of consistent MRI protocols across hospitals, and the frequent artefacts arising in scans from patients who are often restless and confused. Looking at published results, we concluded that improved methods for quantifying intensity changes within the putamen had good potential for development into a clinical tool. However, the apparent gradual reduction in intensity from front to back along the putamen needs to be verified and an appropriate framework for quantifying this validated. In the present study we develop a geometric and intensity model of the putamen with these aims in mind.

2   Methods

2.1   Patients and MRI Scans

27 scans from 20 patients with sCJD, 17 scans from 15 patients with vCJD and 21 scans from 16 non-CJD dementia controls were studied. The diagnosis of CJD was based on international guidelines as definite (with biopsy or autopsy confirmation) or probable (highly likely diagnosis and alternatives excluded). In the controls, further tests and the clinical course of the illness excluded CJD.

The MRI scans were obtained in 16 different hospitals using local clinical protocols. Signal changes within the putamen are best seen in conventional T2 images. Abnormal signal in deep nuclei in CJD may be more conspicuous in diffusion-weighted images [7, 8] and/ or T2 images that are modified to render free fluid dark (often referred to as "FLAIR", fluid-attenuated inversion-recovery T2) [9]. However, there is great variation in acquisition protocols for the latter sequences; for example, FLAIR images are often acquired in the coronal plane, which is unfavourable for analysis of most of the deep nuclei, and diffusion images are often not included at all in routine clinical scans. Furthermore, neither demonstrates the anatomical boundary of the putamen well. T1 weighted images potentially provide the best spatial resolution, but do not show signal abnormalities in CJD, and often do not provide sufficient contrast to show the boundary of the putamen clearly. Therefore, we develop our model of the putamen using T2. In the plane of acquisition, spatial resolution is good (usually about 1 × 1 mm) but slice thickness is large (usually 5 mm) and our model represents the signal gradient in the axial plane only. The best axial slice passing through the whole putamen was manually selected, so that superior and inferior slices that might be affected by partial volume errors were excluded.

2.2   Segmentation and Within-Patient Co-registration

Most automated intensity-based segmentation methods perform poorly with the putamen, reflecting the changing intensities within the structure in normals as well as CJD patients. Atlas-based segmentation has produced promising results [14, 15], but close inspection of boundary localisation shows significant inaccuracies. With clinical MRI scans, we found different MRI sequences were needed to allow confident localisation of different parts of the boundary of one putamen. We therefore performed rigid co-registration of all scans from a single patient to each other and displayed T2, proton density (Fig. 1(a) and (b)) and T1 sequences simultaneously with a linked cursor. Boundaries were drawn manually using MeVisLab [10] (Fig. 1(c)). Quadratic curves were then fitted to the lateral and medial boundaries, and straight lines to the anterior and short posterior borders (Fig. 1(d)). Key landmarks were defined as the intersections of these lines, and the midpoints of the anterior and medial borders. Intermediate landmarks were added at equal arc length along the medial and lateral borders. A skeleton representing the curved long axis of the putamen was derived from the lateral and medial borders and also fitted by a quadratic curve.

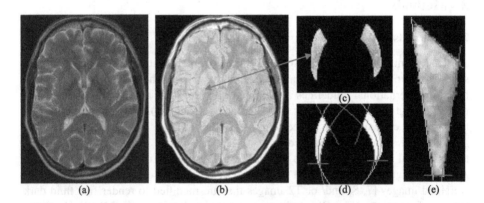

Fig 1. Axial images from one patient. Standard display convention, with anterior at top, patient right on image left etc. Left, (a): T2 weighted, showing gradient most clearly. Centre left, (b): proton density, giving best view of boundary in this patient. Centre right upper, (c): segmented putamen with T2 intensities. Centre right lower, (d): fitted lines and curves for boundaries. The posterior boundary is constrained to be horizontal. Intersections give the main landmarks for co-registration. Right, (e): right putamen warped to geometric model shape; medial and lateral boundaries and skeleton are straightened, and skeleton becomes vertical; grey values are T2 intensities from original image

2.3   The Putamen Model: Spatial and Intensity Normalisation

Preliminary analyses of the intensity changes within the putamen confirmed the visual impression that the main intensity gradient follows the skeleton. We therefore defined the geometry of the model shape so that the skeleton and medial and lateral boundaries were straightened. For some putamens, the posterior part tapers to a tip and a triangle would be a good model. However, in some cases there is a posterior border of significant width, and we truncated the posterior corner of the triangle to define a quadrilateral model shape as shown in Figs. 1(e) and 2. All putamens were co-registered by warping using a thin-plate spline algorithm so that the landmarks exactly corresponded [11, 12].

There is a wide range of absolute intensities between scanners. Intensities were normalised by calculating the within-patient average of the pixel values (left and right putamens combined), and then offsetting each pixel value by the difference between the within-patient average and the global averages across all patients. Note that this linear offset does not affect the gradient magnitude or direction of changes within the putamen.

3   Results

Figure 3 shows images of the model for all patients combined, sCJD, vCJD and controls. Each pixel is the average normalised intensity in the specific group, with left and right putamens combined after reflecting the left model. A gradient of reducing intensity from front to back can be seen clearly in the middle part of the putamen, and appears greater in sCJD than in vCJD or controls. At the posterior end there is a distinct brighter section again. Visually, the main changes were in the longitudinal direction. This was confirmed by analysis of the principal direction of intensity changes, by fitting a plane to the intensity values and projecting the parameters to a sphere; the transverse (i.e. medial-to-lateral changes were inconsistent and the main discrimination was in the longitudinal direction. To reduce dimensions, further

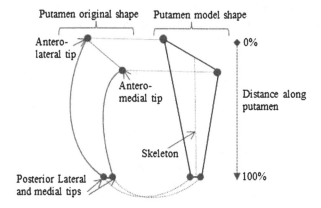

Fig. 2. Putamen model geometry

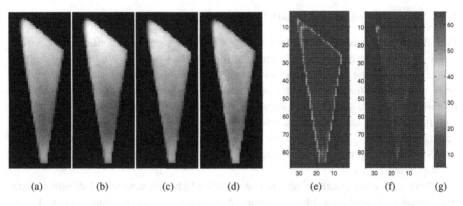

Fig. 3. Images of the model, combining left and right putamens. Grey scale shows group averages. Four images to left of figure use same grey scale of image intensities; from left to right: (a): all patients; (b): sCJD; (c): vCJD; (d): controls. Images to right of figure: (e) standard deviation of intensity values across all patients. (f) standard deviation of intensity values across all patients with 2 pixels boundary removed. (g) standard deviation scale

analyses were carried out by averaging intensities along each line orthogonal to the skeleton and the one-dimensional variation of this mean intensity along the putamen from anterior to posterior was examined.

The variability in different parts of the putamen was examined within groups, and all were similar to the average across all patients shown in Fig. 3, right side. The intensities around the border show a wide variation in values that mainly reflect partial volume effects, and a 2-pixel shell was removed for the further intensity analyses. The bright section at the posterior end of the putamen, which is not arte-factual, is very variable between patients; the posterior 25 % was excluded from the gradient analyses.

The intensities around the border show increased variation in values (Fig. 3(e)) that reflects partial volume effects and a 2-pixel shell was removed for intensity analyses. As mentioned earlier, the largest component of the gradient of intensity change was longitudinal, so further analyses were carried out by averaging the intensities along lines orthogonal to the skeleton i.e. along horizontal lines in the model, generating a single intensity value at each point along the skeleton. Results are presented in the following graphs.

Figure 4 summarises the findings. At the front, there is a rise to an initial peak at 10–15 % along the putamen. Further back, from about 15 % to 70 %, there is a long smooth section, giving way to a brighter section at the posterior end, confirming the visual appearances shown in Fig. 3. To quantify the smooth changes we analysed the central section from 10 % to 65 % and fitted a straight line as shown in Fig. 5. The slopes are highly significant. Furthermore, analysis of covariance showed that there is a highly significant difference in gradient magnitude between sCJD and non-CJD dementia controls (p < 0.0098), while the difference between vCJD and controls was not significant.

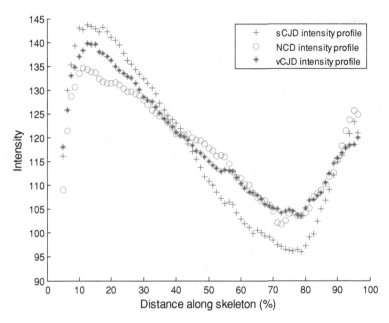

Fig. 4. Graphs of intensity as a function of distance along the skeleton. Each value is the average of intensities along a line orthogonal to the skeleton. Red: average of sCJD group; blue: average of vCJD group; green: average of non-CJD dementia controls (Color figure online)

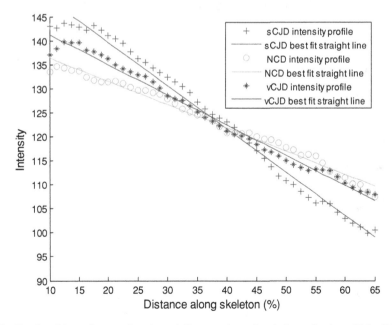

Fig. 5. Graphs of intensity as a function of distance along the skeleton for the middle (10 % to 65 %) section

3.1 Non-parametric Classification

For discrimination between sCJD on the one hand and controls or vCJD on the other, a gradient threshold must be defined; the lower the threshold (in magnitude), the more sensitive the test will be for sCJD but the lower the specificity. For each gradient threshold, we run the test such that for each scan if the magnitude of either the left or right putamen gradient is higher than the gradient threshold, it is a diagnosis of sCJD; otherwise it is a diagnosis of non-CJD dementia. And then we calculated the corresponding sensitivity and specificity. We show this as a graph in Fig. 6. A threshold of -0.8 gives equal sensitivity and specificity values (79 %) and confirms good performance of the test in discriminating between sCJD on the one hand and non-CJD dementia controls or vCJD on the other.

3.2 Logistic Regression Based Classification

The calculated right and left putamen gradients (PG_R and PG_L) were input as two separate variables to the logistic regression procedure to calculate the probability, p, of sCJD diagnosis.

$$\text{logit(p)} = \ln\left[\frac{p}{1-p}\right], \text{and logit(p)} = \beta_0 + \beta_1 * PG_R + \beta_2 * PG_L$$

For the 50 % probability cut-off threshold, the sensitivity was 84 % and specificity 70 %, with an overall accuracy of 78 %.

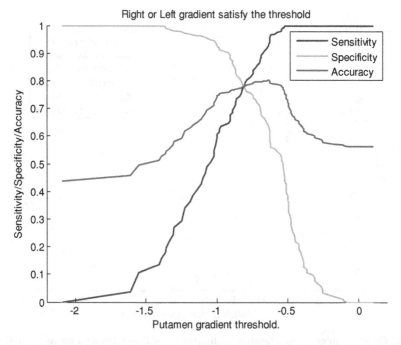

Fig. 6. Plots of sensitivity (blue), specificity (green), and accuracy (red) versus gradient threshold to distinguish between sCJD and non-CJD dementia controls (Color figure online)

4 Discussion

We have developed a model framework to represent the putamen, one of the basal ganglia (deep grey matter nuclei) in the cerebrum, which is known to show abnormal signal intensities in a high proportion of sCJD patients. Most previous work on analysis of intensity abnormalities has focused on average intensities in a region of interest. By dividing the putamen into (arbitrary) parts, significant differences have been confirmed. However, the putamen is unusual in that visually there appears to be a smooth gradient of intensity change within the structure, and in the present work we developed a framework for analysing this systematically. We chose a simple geometric shape to represent the putamen as a straightened object with its skeleton vertical, which is convenient because the main intensity changes occur along this direction. Because the gradient uses within-structure variation, there is an implicit intensity normalisation which helps to overcome the problems of wide variation in intensity values obtained from different scanners.

The averaged model reveals interesting changes of intensity within the putamen that are visible in all patient groups. The smoothly decreasing central part of the putamen is well described by a linear fit (Fig. 5), and the gradient of the line enables good discrimination between sCJD and controls, and also between sCJD and variant CJD. While more complex algebraic models to cover more of the putamen could be designed, individual patient data are very noisy and we suspect that the increased number of parameters to be fitted will limit the usefulness of a more complex approach.

In diagnostic tests where a threshold has to be set to discriminate between groups, there is naturally a pay-off between sensitivity and specificity. An ROC curve can be used to show the relationship between sensitivity and specificity but does not make the changing threshold values explicit. Our plot (Fig. 6) shows the threshold values used and also provides all the information contained in a conventional ROC curve. Depending on the clinical context, the threshold can be adjusted to prioritise either sensitivity or specificity.

There have been advances in other types of diagnostic test in CJD, particularly in the cerebrospinal fluid [13]. However, obtaining the fluid is slightly invasive and is not carried out as an early part of investigation of this type of patient. MRI on the other hand should be obtained in all patients, and more robust methods of flagging possible CJD would have wide clinical applicability. As a screening test our approach could use a lower threshold which would give a higher sensitivity to indicate the need for more invasive tests; the lower specificity would be perfectly acceptable in such a context. In this paper our clinical data are preliminary, and the stated figures are examples rather than definite clinical advice. We are preparing a larger database of patients which will allow fuller clinical evaluation and we will compare the gradient method with other MRI indices.

Acknowledgements. This work was supported by an NHS R&D grant [East Kent Hospitals University Trust].

References

1. Tschampa, H.J., Kallenberg, K., Urbach, H., Meissner, B., Nicolay, C., Kretzschmar, H.A., Knauth, M., Zerr, I.: MRI in the diagnosis of sporadic Creutzfeldt-Jakob disease: a study on inter-observer agreement. Brain **128**, 2026–2033 (2005)
2. Kallenberg, K., Schulz-Schaeffer, W.J., Jastrow, U., et al.: Creutzfeldt-Jakob disease: comparative analysis of MR imaging sequences. Am. J. Neuroradiol. **27**, 1459–1462 (2006)
3. Coulthard, A., Hall, K., English, P.T.: Quantitative analysis of MRI signal intensity in new variant Creutzfeldt-Jakob disease. Brit. J. Radiol. **72**, 742–748 (1999)
4. Fulbright, R.K., Kingsley, P.B., Guo, X., et al.: The imaging appearance of Creutzfeldt-Jakob disease caused by the E200K mutation. Magn. Reson. Imag. **24**, 1121–1129 (2006)
5. Linguraru, M.G., Ayache, N., Bardinet, E., et al.: Differentiation of sCJD and vCJD forms by automated analysis of Basal Gagnlia intensity distribution in multisequence MRI of the brain - definition and evaluation of new MRI-based rations. IEEE Trans. Med. Imag. **25**, 1052–1067 (2006)
6. Hojjat, A., Collie, D., Colchester, A.C.F.: The putamen intensity gradient in CJD diagnosis. In: Dohi, T., Kikinis, R. (eds.) MICCAI 2002, Part I. LNCS, vol. 2488, pp. 524–531. Springer, Heidelberg (2002)
7. Murata, T., Shiga, Y., Higano, S., et al.: Conspicuity and evolution of lesions in Creutzfeldt-Jakob disease at diffusion-weighted imaging. Am. J. Neuroradiol. **23**, 1164–1172 (2002)
8. Romano, A., Bozzao, A., Tisei, P., et al.: Emerging patterns of diffusion, perfusion-weighted MRI and spectroscopy in Creutzfeldt-Jacob disease. Neuroradiol. J. **20**, 56–60 (2007)
9. Collie, D.A., Summers, D.M., Sellar, R.J., et al.: Diagnosing variant Creutzfeldt-Jakob disease with the pulvinar sign: MR imaging findings in 86 Neuropathologically confirmed cases. Am. J. Neuroradiol. **24**, 1560–1569 (2003)
10. Heckel, F., Konrad, O., Karl Hahn, H., et al.: Interactive 3D medical image segmentation with energy-minimizing implicit functions. Comput. Graph. **35**, 275–287 (2011)
11. Bookstein, F.L.: Principal Warps: thin-plate splines and the decomposition of deformations. IEEE Trans. Pattern Anal. Mach. Intell. **11**, 567–585 (1989)
12. Schnabel, J.A., Rueckert, D., Quist, M., Blackall, J.M., Castellano-Smith, A.D., Hartkens, T., Penney, G.P., Hall, W.A., Liu, H., Truwit, C.L., Gerritsen, F.A., Hill, D.L.G., Hawkes, David J.: A generic framework for non-rigid registration based on non-uniform multi-level free-form deformations. In: Niessen, Wiro J., Viergever, M.A. (eds.) MICCAI 2001. LNCS, vol. 2208, pp. 573–581. Springer, Heidelberg (2001)
13. McGuire, L.I., Peden, A.H., Orrú, C.D., et al.: Real time quaking-induced conversion analysis of cerebrospinal fluid in sporadic Creutzfeldt-Jakob disease. Ann. Neurol. **72**, 278–285 (2012)
14. Aljabar, P., Heckemann, R.A., Hammers, A., et al.: Multi-atlas based segmentation of brain images: atlas selection and its effect on accuracy. Neuroimage **46**, 726–738 (2009)
15. Cabezas, M., Oliver, A., Lladó, X., et al.: A review of atlas-based segmentation for magnetic resonance brain images. Comput. Methods Programs Biomed. **104**, e158–e177 (2011)

Inter-slice Correspondence for 2D Ultrasound-Guided Procedures

Matthew Toews$^{(\boxtimes)}$, Alexandra J. Golby, and William M. Wells III

Brigham and Women's Hospital, Harvard Medical School, Boston, USA
{mt,sw}@bwh.harvard.edu, AGOLBY@partners.org

Abstract. This paper reports on a new computational methodology, inter-slice correspondence (ISC), for robustly aligning sets of 2D ultrasound (US) slices during image-guided medical procedures. Correspondences are derived from distinctive, local scale-invariant features, which are used in one-to-many matching of US slices in near real-time despite out-of-plane rotation, in addition to global in-plane similarity transforms, occlusion, missing tissue, US plane mirroring, changes in US probe depth settings. Experiments demonstrate that ISC can align manually-acquired US slices without probe tracking information in the context of image-guided neurosurgery, with an accuracy of 1.3 mm. A novel reconstruction-without-calibration application based on ISC is proposed, where 3D US reconstruction results are very similar to those obtained via traditional phantom-based calibration.

1 Introduction

Freehand ultrasound is a cheap, safe and portable imaging modality for intra-operative guidance and visualization. Although 3D ultrasound sensors exist, 2D probes remain widely used in clinical practice due to their relatively high image quality and low cost [1]. Intraoperative guidance and visualization frequently require relating 2D US slices acquired from a hand-held probe to the 3D patient anatomy. Most published techniques rely heavily on external tracking systems, e.g. optical or electromagnetic, which provide the rigid location and orientation of a tracking target fixed to the US probe for each US image frame [1–4].

Although useful, probe tracking systems have important limitations. Calibration procedures are typically required to transform the US image geometry to that of the tracked probe [2], which involve scanning a specialized phantom every time the image-to-probe geometry may have changed, e.g. following instrument sterilization. Even relatively simple calibration methods [3] require additional equipment, procedures and expertise, complicating the clinical work flow. Loss of calibration or tracking (e.g. due changing US probe depth settings, physical accidents [4], loss of line-of-sight) during a medical procedure result in image-guidance failure. Tracker-free matching of US data [5] offers a potential online solution, however current systems do not address out-of-plane alignment. Speckle decorrelation techniques can potentially measure out-of-plane motion [6–8], how-ever practical applications based on manually-acquired data in a clinical setting remain challenging.

M. Erdt et al. (Eds.): CLIP 2013, LNCS 8361, pp. 143–150, 2014.
DOI: 10.1007/978-3-319-05666-1_18, © Springer International Publishing Switzerland 2014

This paper proposes a new computational methodology in order to reduce the reliance of US-guidance on probe tracking systems: inter-slice correspondence (ISC). ISC identifies local image correspondences between 2D US slices acquired from different probe positions, robustly and in near real-time, despite out-of-plane rotations, in-plane translation, orientation and scale changes. Experiments demonstrate that ISCs can be accurately computed between manually acquired US slices during neurosurgery without probe tracking. A novel application of ISC is proposed: US volume reconstruction without calibration, where reconstruction results are similar to those obtained via phantom-based calibration.

2   Inter-slice Correspondence

Inter-slice correspondence (ISC) aims to map image structure from a US slice to homologous structure in a sequence of previously acquired 2D US slices. Although ISC can be used in conjunction with probe tracking information, for example in the 3D reconstruction method proposed in the following section, it is achieved without probe tracking information. To be effective in an arbitrary interventional setting, ISC must account for a significant degree of deformed or missing tissue, e.g. in the case of resection, in addition to in-plane geometrical variations such as such as translation, rotation and scaling, e.g. in case of variation in probe position or depth settings. Most importantly, ISC must account for out-of-plane geometrical variations, as US data are generally acquired from different 3D slices through the patient anatomy. To this end, ISC operates by identifying correspondences between informative local patterns or features that can be reliably localized in multiple, approximately intersecting US planes.

ISC makes use of local scale-invariant image features, distinctive image patterns that can be automatically extracted in each US slice in a manner independent of in-plane translation, orientation and scale changes [9,10]. A feature $f = \{\bar{u}, \theta, \sigma, \bar{a}\}$ is an oriented image patch described geometrically by 2D pixel location $\bar{u} = \{u, v\}$, orientation θ and scale σ, along with a local intensity descriptor $\bar{a}$ used for computing correspondence. A number of scale-invariant feature extractors exist, we adopt the computationally efficient 'SURF' algorithm [10]. Briefly, salient image regions $(\bar{u}, \theta, \sigma)$ are identified based on the local Hessian determinant, and local intensity is encoded via a 64-element descriptor of $\bar{a}$ of Haar wavelet responses.

Robust feature correspondence has been the focus of extensive research in the context of computer vision, where techniques such RANSAC and the Hough transform are commonly used to identify correct feature matches between pairs of projective images, for example [9–11]. The context of US data bears distinct challenges, however, and these techniques cannot be applied directly. To illustrate, in the context of projective image data, the same 3D point is generally observable in images acquired from different sensor geometrical configurations, i.e. camera viewpoints, and relatively dense correspondences can be identified via pair-wise image matching. In contrast, US data are not formed via projection but rather as slices through 3D space, and the same 3D point cannot generally be observed as slices generally do not pass through precisely the same point. Thus whereas relatively dense correspondences can be identified between an arbitrary pair of projective images, e.g. photographs of the same scene, valid correspondences generally do not exist between an arbitrary pair of US images.

ISC thus adopts a novel robust one-to-many correspondence technique, that aims to identify approximately correct matches between a new US image and an entire sequence of previously acquired US slices, as illustrated in Fig. 1. Let I and $\bar{I}'$ represent sets of features extracted in a new US image and in a sequence of previously acquired (i.e. prior or training) US slices, respectively. ISC identifies correspondences (f, f') between all features $f \in I$ and some feature $f' \in \bar{I}'$, by pairing each f with a nearest neighbor (NN) f' based on the Euclidean distance of local feature intensity descriptors $\|\bar{a}, \bar{a}'\|$. Fast approximate NN techniques operate in $O(N \log N)$ computation complexity in the number of training features $N = |\bar{I}'|$, e.g. using the k-d tree data structure [12]. An additional US-related consideration is the case of mirrored image correspondence due to lateral probe flipping, this can be accounted for efficiently by mirroring the geometry and appearance descriptor elements of $f \in I$ prior to correspondence.

Many ISCs are spurious and noisy, and robust estimation is required to identify a reduced set of valid correspondences. The geometrical mapping between ISC arising from multiple US slices is modeled as a global in-plane similarity transform followed by local feature-specific variations. Intuitively, the similarity transform coarsely approximates global image pattern variation between nearby slices in the 3D world, about which variations due to out-of-plane rotation, non-linear tissue deformation, occlusion, etc., are approximated as locally linear via individual correspondences. The Hough transform is used to identify a globally optimal similarity transform, as follows. Let $\Psi = \{d\bar{u}, d\theta, d\sigma\}$ represent the 2D translation, rotation and scaling parameters of an in-plane similarity transform mapping the geometry of f' to that of f. The set $C(\Psi) = \{ (f, f') :$

$$\text{NN}(a, a') \ \wedge \ \|\bar{u}, \bar{u}' + d\bar{u}\|/\sigma \leq \epsilon_u \ \wedge \ |\log \sigma' d\sigma/\sigma| \leq \epsilon_\sigma \ \wedge \ |\theta - \theta' + d\theta| \leq \epsilon_\theta$$

$\}$ contains the inliers of Ψ, i.e. all nearest neighbor correspondences $\text{NN}(f, f')$ such that the differences in scale-normalized location, scale and orientation of feature f and f' transformed by Ψ are within thresholds $(\epsilon_u, \epsilon_\sigma, \epsilon_\theta)$. An optimal transform $\Psi^* = \operatorname*{argmax}_\Psi |C(\Psi)|$ maximizing the cardinality or inlier count of $C(\Psi)$ is identified by testing candidate transforms generated by each correspondence, and the final set of ISC inliers is $C(\Psi^*)$. Thresholds are set empirically, higher values allow a high degree of ISC deformation while increasing the incorrect ISC rate. Values of $(\epsilon_u = 3/4, \epsilon_\sigma = \log 1.5, \epsilon_\theta = 20°)$ are used here for all experiments. A final constraint requires correspondences to occur within sequential frames of $\bar{I}'$, under the assumption of a smoothly varying US probe acquisition trajectory.

The accuracy of ISC with respect to ground truth is evaluated in the context of neurosurgery, with two freehand US sweeps of the same human brain acquired prior to major resection. The BITE data set is used [4], where a calibrated probe tracking system provides a ground truth mapping between US pixel coordinates

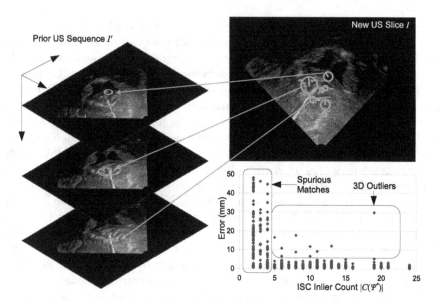

Fig. 1. Illustrating inter-slice correspondences via scale-invariant feature (green circles) from a new US slice (upper right) to multiple US slices in a prior sequence (left). A graph of 3D ISC error vs. ISC inlier count (lower right) reveals low error for inlier counts greater than 4, with the exception of a small number of 3D outliers.

to 3D anatomical locations. Images are 640×480 with $0.2 \, \text{mm}$ resolution, each producing ≈ 800 features. One sweep is arbitrarily chosen as the prior sequence $\bar{I}'$ (240 slices), and ISC is performed to each slice I of a second sweep (144 slices). Figure 1 graphs the error (Euclidean distance) for ground truth 3D locations of ISC correspondences. Error is high for slices where $|C(\Psi^*) < 5|$, these are generally incorrectly aligned due to insufficient overlap of US content. This is expected, since the volumetric overlap of sweep 2 with sweep 1 here is $\approx 78\,\%$. Error is low for slices where $|C(\Psi^*)| \geq 5$, with the exception of a small number (2.2 %) of *3D Outliers*, i.e. coincidental correspondences that are in-plane inliers but incorrect outliers in 3D. In total, 41 % of testing slices I result $|C(\Psi^*)| \geq 5$, with an average ISC error of 1.3 mm. Note that the number of ISC inliers can be used to identify US frames with no valid correspondence. 3D outliers have a negligible impact on volume reconstruction in the following section.

3   US Volume Reconstruction Without Calibration

US Volume reconstruction is commonly used for visualizing 3D patient anatomy from a set of tracked, freehand 2D US frames. Reconstruction typically requires estimating the US image-to-probe transform via a specialized calibration procedure and apparatus [2]. Calibration-free methods for computing the image-to-probe transform have been proposed, however they come with limitations (e.g. no recovery of out-of-plane rotation [13] or scaling parameters [14]), or require a specific US acquisition protocol (e.g. two image sequences separated by a 90° out-of-plane rotation about a fixed 3D point [14]).

ISC allows calibration-free reconstruction from relatively unconstrained US sweeps through arbitrary, textured tissues. Let $\bar{x}_i = [x_i, y_i, z_i, 1]^T$ represent the location of a 3D point in the world in homogenous coordinates, and let $\bar{u}_i = [u_i, v_i, 0, 1]^T$ represent the pixel location of the same point within a 2D US image. Points $\bar{u}_i$ and $\bar{x}_i$ are related by the following equation:

$$\bar{x}_i = T_w T_p T_s \bar{u}_i, \tag{1}$$

where T_w, T_p and T_s are 4×4 homogenous transform matrices. T_w is a rigid transform from the US probe to the 3D world, typically provided for each US image by the tracking mechanism. $T_s = \text{diag}[s_u, s_v, 1, 1]$ is a diagonal scaling matrix converting US spatial units (pixels) to world distance units (mm). Scaling parameters (s_u, s_v) may in principle be provided by the US system, however they vary with changes in US settings such as depth, and are treated as unknown here. Finally, T_p is the unknown rigid transform from the US image plane to the US probe, with six intrinsic parameters: three rotation angles and three coordinate translations. For simplicity, let $T_{ps} = T_p T_s$ represent the unknown image-to-probe transform matrix.

The goal of 3D reconstruction here is to determine the unknown T_{ps} from ISCs identified between US slices. Let $(\bar{u}_i, \bar{u}_i')$ represent corresponding US image points, i.e. the locations of the same 3D point x_i observed in two different US images. From Eq. (1), corresponding points $\bar{u}_i$ and $\bar{u}_i'$ are related via the following equation:

$$T_w' T_{ps} \bar{u}_i' = T_w T_{ps} \bar{u}_i + \eta_i, \tag{2}$$

where η_i is assumed to be zero-mean Gaussian noise. Thus given a set of N correspondences $\{(\bar{u}_1, \bar{u}_1'), \ldots, (\bar{u}_i, \bar{u}_i'), \ldots, (\bar{u}_N, \bar{u}_N')\}$, the optimal matrix T_{ps}^* minimizing the squared reconstruction error of corresponding points in the 3D world becomes:

$$T_{ps}^* = \underset{T_{ps}}{\text{argmin}} \left\{ \sum_{i=1}^{N} ||T_w' T_{ps} \bar{u}_i' - T_w T_{ps} \bar{u}_i||^2 \right\}, \tag{3}$$

T_{ps} is a scaled rigid transform defined by eight intrinsic parameters: a 3D displacement vector $\bar{d} = \{d_1, d_2, d_3\}$, two positive scaling factors (s_u, s_v) treated here as unconstrained values in the log domain $(\log(s_u), \log(s_v))$, and three rotation parameters constrained by the orthonormality requirements of a 3×3 rotation matrix. Rotation parameter constraints complicate optimization of Eq. (3), here we adopt a Rodrigues parameterization in which a 3D rotation is represented as scalar angular rotation about a 3D axis. Specifically, a 3D vector of unconstrained values $\bar{\omega} = \{\omega_1, \omega_2, \omega_3\}$ is adopted, where the unit vector $\frac{\bar{\omega}}{||\bar{\omega}||}$ defines the rotation axis and the the norm $||\bar{\omega}||$ defines the rotation angle.

Optimization thus seeks to identify a parameter vector $\{\log(s_u), \log(s_v), \bar{d}, \bar{\omega}\}$ minimizing Eq. (3). A variety of non-linear optimization methods could be brought to bear, here we adopt the Nelder-Mead simplex method [15] which does not require explicit gradient computation and converges reliably in optimization scenarios involving small numbers of parameters. Additionally, rather than minimize the squared error over all correspondences, optimization considers the squared error of the 75 % of correspondences with minimum error, in order to reduce the influence of potential 3D outlier ISCs.

Reconstruction is tested using two 900-slice tracked US sequences of the brain, acquired prior to major resection in the context of neurosurgery. The sequences are acquired via arbitrary sweeps along similar trajectories, consisting of translation and minor 3D rotations. ISCs are identified between slices in different sequences as in Sect. 2, then used to estimate T_{ps} via optimization of Eq. (3). An important note is that ISCs must be identified over a degree of out-of-plane rotation in order avoid degeneracy in estimating T_{ps}. For comparison purposes, T_{ps} is also estimated via a standard wire phantom-based calibration procedure (see PLUS perk.cs.queensu.ca). The discrepancy between T_{ps} parameters for the two methods is low: scale parameters (isotropic here) differ by $0.1045 - 0.1064$ or $\approx 1.8\,\%$, rotation direction cosines differ by $2.8°, 2.4°, 1.6°$. The reconstruction error for 3D correspondences following estimation of T_{ps} is 0.35 mm. Volumes are reconstructed from one tracked 900-frame sequence using a simple trilinear interpolation method, using T_{ps} obtained via the calibration-free ISC method and standard calibration. These are shown in Fig. 2, note the high degree of visual similarity.

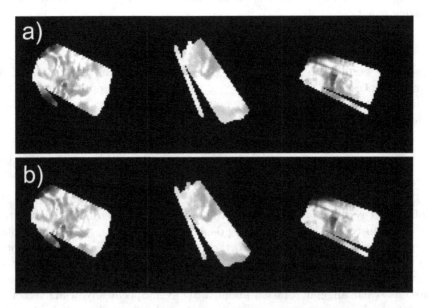

Fig. 2. Axial, sagittal and coronal cross sections of reconstructed US volumes: (a) calibration-free ISC and (b) standard calibration-based. Note the visual similarity.

4   Discussion

Inter-slice correspondence (ISC) is presented as a novel method for aligning 2D ultrasound data without external probe tracking. Correspondences can be identified across a wide range of variations, including out-of-plane rotation, and exhibit relatively low error (1.3 mm) with respect to ground truth. Correspondence failure can be detected, e.g. in the case where no valid correspondence exists, by the number of ISC inliers. ISC is efficient; an unoptimized C++ implementation runs at approximately 3 frames per second on a 2.5 GHz processor for 640×480 pixel US slices. Computation time is largely due to feature extraction and could be reduced via parallelized GPU processing.

The primary potential for ISC is in increasing the robustness of 2D US-guidance by reducing the dependency on external tracking. This is demonstrated in a novel calibration-free US volume reconstruction formulation based on ICSs, where results are similar to those obtained by a phantom-based calibration procedure with an average reconstruction error of 0.35 mm. Other potential applications could include automatic verification of calibration during a procedure or navigation and visualization in the case of tracking or calibration failure, these are left for future work.

Several considerations regarding ISC should be noted. The anatomy of interest must contain distinctive, localizable image structure from which distinctive features can be extracted. Qualitatively, we have noted ISC to be effective in US of various organs, including muscle. ISCs cannot be computed if the degree out-of-plane rotation between slices is too great, this breakdown point will be investigated. Future work will include quantifying ground-truth ISC accuracy in intraoperative data, investigating ISC for the purpose of online navigation for image guidance in neurosurgery and in other domains (e.g. abdomen), improvements to tracker-less visualization (e.g. deformable tumor contour alignment) and developing a probabilistic model of ISC.

Acknowledgements. This work was supported by NIH grants R01CA138419 and P41EB015898 and P41EB015902.

References

1. Prager, R.W., Ijaz, U.Z., Gee, A.H., Treece, G.M.: Three-dimensional ultrasound imaging. J. Eng. Med. **224**, 192–223 (2010)
2. Mercier, L., Lang, T., Lindsesth, F., Collins, D.L.: A review of calibration techniques for freehand 3-d ultrasound systems. Ultrasound Med. Biol. **31**(4), 449–471 (2005)
3. Khamene, A., Sauer, F.: A novel phantom-less spatial and temporal ultrasound calibration method. In: Duncan, J.S., Gerig, G. (eds.) MICCAI 2005. LNCS, vol. 3750, pp. 65–72. Springer, Heidelberg (2005)
4. Mercier, L., Del Maestro, R.F., Petrecca, K., Araujo, D., Haegelen, C., Collins, D.L.: Online database of clinical mr and ultrasound images of brain tumors. Med. Phys. **39**, 3253 (2012)

5. Kwitt, R., Vasconcelos, N., Razzaque, S., Aylward, S.: Recognition in ultrasound videos: where am i? In: Ayache, N., Delingette, H., Golland, P., Mori, K. (eds.) MICCAI 2012, Part III. LNCS, vol. 7512, pp. 83–90. Springer, Heidelberg (2012)
6. James Housden, R., Gee, A.H., Treece, G.M., Prager, R.W.: Sensorless reconstruction of freehand 3d ultrasound data. In: Larsen, R., Nielsen, M., Sporring, J. (eds.) MICCAI 2006. LNCS, vol. 4191, pp. 356–363. Springer, Heidelberg (2006)
7. Laporte, C., Arbel, T.: Learning to estimate out-of-plane motion in ultrasound imagery of real tissue. MIA 15, 202–213 (2011)
8. Afsham, N., Najafi, M., Abolmaesumi, P., Rohling, R.: Out-of-plane motion estimation based on a rician-inverse gaussian model of rf ultrasound signals: speckle tracking without fully developed speckle. In: Proceedings of SPIE, vol. 8320, p. 832017-1 (2012)
9. Lowe, D.G.: Distinctive image features from scale-invariant keypoints. IJCV 60(2), 91–110 (2004)
10. Bay, H., Tuytelaars, T., Gool, L.V.: Surf: speeded up robust features. CVIU 110(3), 346–359 (2008)
11. Mirota, D., Uneri, A., Schafer, S., Nithiananthan, S., Reh, D., Ishii, M., Gallia, G., Taylor, R., Hager, G., Siewerdsen, J.: Evaluation of a system for high-accuracy 3d image-based registration of endoscopic video to c-arm cone-beam ct for image-guided skull base surgery. IEEE TMI 32(7), 1215–1226 (2013)
12. Muja, M., Lowe, D.G.: Fast approximate nearest neighbors with automatic algorithm configuration. In: International Conference on Computer Vision, pp. 331–340 (2009)
13. Boctor, E., Iordachita, I., Fichtinger, G., Hager, G.: Ultrasound self-calibration. In: SPIE Medical Imaging, pp. 61412N–61412N (2006)
14. Wein, W., Khamene, A.: Image-based method for in-vivo freehand ultrasound calibration. In: SPIE Medical Imaging, vol. 6920 (2008)
15. Nelder, J.A., Mead, R.: A simplex method for function minimization. Comput. J. 7, 308–313 (1965)

First Clinical Experience with BMD Assessment in Vertebrae Using Dual-Energy CT

Stefan Wesarg[1]($\boxtimes$), Julian Wichmann[2], Christian Booz[2], Marius Erdt[3],
Konstantinos Kafchitsas[4], and M. Fawad Khan[2]

[1] Fraunhofer Institute for Computer Graphics Research, Darmstadt, Germany
stefan.wesarg@igd.fraunhofer.de
[2] Institute for Diagnostic and Interventional Radiology, Goethe University,
Frankfurt am Main, Germany
[3] Fraunhofer IDM@NTU, Singapore, Singapore
[4] Clinic and Polyclinic for Orthopedics and Orthopedic Surgery,
Universitätsmedizin Mainz, Mainz, Germany

Abstract. Dual-energy CT (DECT) can be performed with state-of-the-art dual-source CT (DSCT) scanners and allows for assessing bone mineral density (BMD). In this work, we present first clinical experience with in vivo BMD assessment of vertebrae based on DECT data which has been acquired with a state-of-the-art DSCT scanner in the clinical routine. In contrast to previous work where we did *in vitro* tests of our method, we apply it her for the first time to *in vivo* data and prove the feasibility of our technique in a clinical setting. For 25 patients, DXA as well as DECT data have been acquired and BMD of vertebrae was assessed. Advantages of DECT are its 3D capabilities allowing to compute the spatial BMD distribution and to focus the examination on the trabecular bone. Correlation between both imaging techniques regarding the averaged BMD values per vertebra are only moderate.

Keywords: Bone mineral density · Dual-energy CT · Osteoporosis

1 Introduction

Lowered bone mineral density (BMD) is an indicator for reduced bone stability [11]. This might lead to *osteoporosis* where the fracture risk is increased due to a deterioration of the micro-structure of the trabecular bone. This constituent is the inner part of many bony structures like vertebrae who have an additional outer shell – the cortical bone. Having a higher metabolic activity [3], the trabecular bone of vertebrae is more affected by a decrease of BMD than the cortical bone. The latter sometimes compensates this lowered BMD to some extent by becoming locally more dense.

Thus, from the clinical point of view it is desirable to have a means to examine both, trabecular and cortical bone independently. However, the currently used

M. Erdt et al. (Eds.): CLIP 2013, LNCS 8361, pp. 151–159, 2014.
DOI: 10.1007/978-3-319-05666-1_19, © Springer International Publishing Switzerland 2014

standard imaging modality for BMD assessment is dual-energy X-ray absorptiometry (DXA) which provides 2D projection images of the bone - e.g., vertebrae [2,8]. There, the measured intensity represents the combined absorption of both vertebral constituents. And a separation of both contributions is not possible. A method for a localized assessment of BMD is quantitative computed tomography (qCT) [1]. This 3D imaging modality allows for a regional analysis of the bone and directly delivers BMD values. This is achieved by placing a calibration phantom in the field-of-view of the CT scanner. The phantom contains substances with known density allowing for a direct determination of BMD values based on the measured intensity in qCT.

In the past years, dual-source computed tomography (DSCT) technology has become available in the clinics. These scanners contain two pairs of X-ray source and detector, respectively [5]. Since both sources can be operated with different energies, dual-energy computed tomography (DECT) can be performed easily. Even though the use of DECT for BMD assessment has been already proposed in the last century [6,7], it has not gained attraction yet despite the availability of DSCT technology.

In a previous publication [10], we presented a method for BMD assessment in vertebrae employing 3D DECT image data. Besides the presentation of our approach, the focus of that work was an *in vitro* evaluation using cadaver specimens. The computed BMD values for the trabecular bone were compared with measurements of pull-out forces applied to screws which have been drilled into the pedicles of the individual vertebrae. We could show that there is a relatively strong correlation between the BMD values and the bone stability derived from the force measurements. In this work, we present the outcome of a first clinical study focusing on BMD assessment based on DECT and using our method. For this, 25 patients underwent DXA and DECT imaging, respectively. Purpose of the study was to investigate the clinical practicability of DECT based BMD assessment doing in vivo tests for the first time and to analyze the data regarding any potential correlation between DXA and DECT measurements.

2   Methods

2.1   Biophysical Model of the Trabecular Bone

As mentioned above, methods for assessing BMD based on DECT have already been proposed in the last century. In a comparative study [9], the approach of Nickoloff et al. [7] performed best. Therefore, it was integrated into our solution. The underlying biophysical model expresses the normalized overall volume of the trabecular bone as the sum of the partial volumes of its constituents – trabecular bone V_{TB}, adipose tissue V_F, and non-adipose tissue V_T:

$$V_{TB} + V_F + V_T = 1. \tag{1}$$

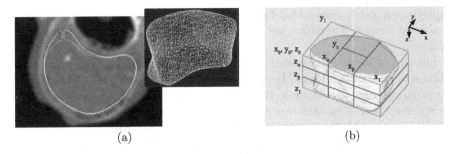

(a)   (b)

Fig. 1. By deforming the template mesh it is adapted to the individual shape of each vertebra. Its adjustable stiffness affects the influence of this deformation to the interaction point's vicinity (a). Subdivision of the trabecular bone mask into 12 segments (b).

The relationship between the measured Hounsfield values χ_{HU}^{low} and χ_{HU}^{high} and the fractional volumes V_{TB} and V_F is given by the following two (manufacturer independent) equations:

$$\chi_{HU}^{low} = (\mu^{low} - \gamma^{low}g) \cdot V_{TB} + (\beta^{low}t - \gamma^{low}g) \cdot V_F + \gamma^{low}g + \delta + \epsilon, \quad (2)$$

$$\chi_{HU}^{high} = (\mu^{high} - \gamma^{high}g) \cdot V_{TB} + (\beta^{high}t - \gamma^{high}g) \cdot V_F + \gamma^{high}g + \delta + \epsilon. \quad (3)$$

here, *low* and *high* stand for the two energies of the DSCT scanner's sources. Typical values are $80\,kV$ and $140\,kV$. Altogether, these are three equations for three unknowns allowing to compute the three fractional volumes. The value of V_{TB} is directly proportional to the BMD of the trabecular bone ρ_{BM} and given as

$$\rho_{BM} = \frac{l \cdot V_{TB}}{1 + \lambda}. \quad (4)$$

The variables in the Eqs. 2 to 4 are energy dependent constants. Their values for different energies can be found in reference [7].

2.2   Labeling of the Trabecular Bone

Since we are interested in the BMD of the trabecular bone, this region has to be delineated in the DECT image data first. Afterwards, the computation of ρ_{BM} can be restricted to these areas considering the intensity values in the low and high energy data sets. In reference [10], we presented two different methods for this labeling – an interactive one as well as an automatic one. For the clinical study presented here, we selected the interactive one [4]. Initial feedback given by the clinical users was that they want to maintain full control over the labeling step, thus favoring the interactive method. Furthermore, our automatic method employing an *Active Shape Model* segmentation was trained with a rather limited number of shapes. Therefore, we could not fully guarantee its robustness and accuracy.

Initially, a mesh representation of a manually segmented trabecular bone region was created using the Marching Cubes algorithm. This mesh was further processed in order to distribute the vertices evenly. It served as a template for the segmentation of an arbitrary vertebra. For this, the clinician has to roughly align the mesh with the image data through translation, rotation, and scaling. Afterwards, the mesh can be locally deformed by pulling the boundaries of the mesh towards the desired position (Fig. 1, *left*). The exerted force at a specific vertex is always propagated to adjacent nodes using a 3D Gaussian. Switching between different scales of the standard deviation σ allows for a variation of the mesh's stiffness. For ensuring that no distortion artifacts occur, an optimization of the point distribution is immediately performed during the adaptation of the mesh. If the user is satisfied with the delineation of the trabecular region, a mask image is created where all voxels inside the resulting mesh are labeled.

2.3   BMD Computation

In order to assess the BMD values inside the defined volume-of-interest (VOI), the two DECT data sets (low and high energy) as well as the generated label volume have to be loaded into our BMD processing tool. There, the user also has to set the energy values for the DECT data and select the basic type of the vertebra (lumbar, thoracic, or cervical) to be analyzed. The latter is necessary for a correct color-coding of the computed BMD values. Reference [12] gives typical BMD values for the different vertebrae obtained through qCT based measurements over a large cohort. The there given average and variance values define the range for the coloring in our software.

Our software performs two different BMD computations. In any case, the computation is always restricted to the labeled region. The first variant is a voxel-wise computation providing the spatial BMD distribution in the considered VOI. For each voxel and its close 3D neighborhood, a Gaussian-weighted intensity value is computed from low and high energy image data (the χ_{HU} in Eqs. 2 and 3). Thus, we obtain a ρ_{BM} value for every voxel in the VOI. For the second variant, we first subdivide the trabecular bone into 12 segments (Fig. 1, *right*). Along the direction of the vertebral column, the vertebra is divided into 3 regions, and each of them further into 4 parts. This segmentation is clinically justified: the left and right part of the vertebra may be regions where during therapy pedicle screws will be drilled in; the BMD distribution close to the vertebral endplates is expected to be different from that of the central region; and ventral as well as dorsal regions should be examined separately. For each segment, the intensity values χ_{HU} are averaged. And one value ρ_{BM} is computed per segment. These 12 values are written to a file for further statistical analysis.

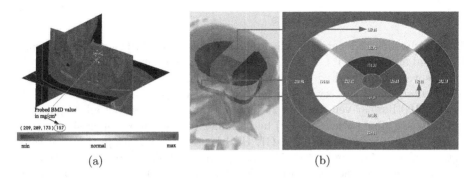

Fig. 2. Visualization of the spatial BMD distribution for a lumbar vertebra employing three orthogonal slices. The density values are mapped to color where the minimum and maximum values depend on the type of vertebra. Direct probing at the position indicated by the cross-hair provides the corresponding BMD value (a). The vertebral body is subdivided into 12 segments. For each of them, a single BMD value is computed and mapped to color. In addition, these values are displayed employing an elliptical plot (b).

2.4 Visualization

For the display of the computed values, we provide the BMD values and show their spatial relationship to other parts of the vertebra. Therefore, we generate an output image I_{BMD} based on the input image data. For voxels lying outside the VOI, we simply copy the intensity values from the low energy image and shift them above 4095, i.e., $I_{BMD} = I_0 + 4096$. The voxels inside the VOI are set to the BMD values. That way, a color transfer function can be defined that provides a standard gray level visualization for the unchanged voxel intensities above 4095 and a color mapping for values ranging from 0 to 4095. Depending on the type of the vertebra, the BMD values are mapped to color employing a perceptually based red-to-blue color map[1]. Here, low density regions appear reddish, areas of normal density white, and high density regions bluish.

The spatial BMD distribution is displayed using three orthogonal planes which can be interactively moved through the image data set. In addition to the color coding of the trabecular bone region, single voxel positions can be probed which causes that the corresponding BMD value is displayed on the screen (Fig. 2, *left*). The values of the 12 segments are displayed employing an elliptical 2D plot. This provides a comprehensive overview over the BMD values in the 12 segments (Fig. 2, *right*). This type of visualization is inspired from cardiology, where a so-called *bull's-eye display* is employed for the display of cardiac parameters. Due to the fact that the vertebral body's cross sectional area is rather elliptical, we adapt the display in our case to an elliptical shape.

---

[1] The color map is taken from http://colorbrewer2.org

2.5 Patients and Image Data

This study included patients who were scheduled for BMD assessment using DXA and an additional CT scan of the abdomen or lumbar spine. Both examinations were performed within an interval of 48 h. Patients with metallic implements after spinal surgery or hip replacements were excluded in this study. A total of 100 lumbar vertebrae in 25 patients were evaluated. Of all 25 patients in this study, nine patients (36 %) had a known history of osteoporosis.

DXA was performed using a GE Healthcare *Lunar Prodigy Advance bone densitometer* (Madison, WI, USA). Images of the lumbar spine (L1-L4) were obtained in anterior-posterior acquisition. For each vertebra, the manufacturer's software automatically calculated BMD values. The DECT examinations in this study were performed using a second generation 128-slice DSCT in dual-energy mode (*Somatom Definition Flash*, Siemens Healthcare, Forchheim, Germany). Both X-ray tubes were operated at different kilo voltage settings (tube A: $140\,kVp$ with Sn filter, $105\,mAs$ per rotation; tube B: $100\,kVp$, $165\,mAs$ per rotation). Image series were acquired in the craniocaudal direction with patients in a supine position and both arms extended above the head. Images were reconstructed with a dedicated dual-energy bone kernel (D70f) and the recorded information of the full gantry rotation (temporal resolution of $280\,ms$) with a slice thickness of $1.5\,mm$ and an increment of $1.0\,mm$.

3 Results

The developed software could easily be used by the clinicians participating in this study. After a short training period, the labeling of the trabecular region employing the interactive template mesh deformation method could be done autonomously. The time needed for the labeling ranged from 2 to $5\,min$ per vertebra. Once the VOI had been defined, the BMD assessment itself run autonomously. On a standard notebook PC, the time needed for processing a complete DECT data set was below $10\,s$. Afterwards, the clinician was presented with the eliptical 12 segments plot and could interactively examine the spatial BMD distribution using the orthogonal plane visualization and probing.

The average DECT-based BMD value computed from all 25 subjects was $0.215\,g/cm^3 \pm 0.049\,g/cm^3$, ranging from $0.131\,g/cm^3$ up to $0.395\,g/cm^3$. Thus, these values correspond well to other studies where BMD was assessed based on qCT data [12]. Regarding DXA, calculated average bone density of L1-L4 was $0.951\,g/cm^2 \pm 0.234\,g/cm^2$, ranging from $0.643\,g/cm^2$ up to $1.641\,g/cm^2$. According to the WHO guidelines, DXA measurements identified seventeen vertebrae (17 %) as osteopenic. Fifty-four (54 %) vertebrae showed an osteoporotic BMD measured by DXA. The correlation between the computed BMD values based on DECT and DXA, respectively, was only moderate (Fig. 3).

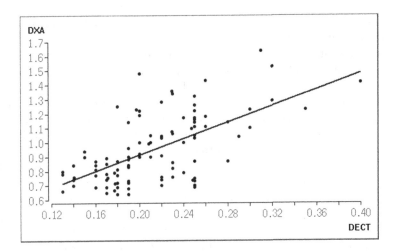

Fig. 3. Correlation between DECT and DXA values. A linear regression has been applied leading to a coefficient of determination $r^2 = 0.3764$.

4   Discussion

We have successfully performed a first clinical study with a novel method for BMD assessment based on DECT. Initially, the software had been tested only in vitro using cadaver specimens [10]. Here, a pilot clinical study showed that DECT-based in vivo BMD assessment is feasible and allows for segmented display of 3D trabecular BMD distribution of the lumbar spine. In addition, the clinicians involved in this work stated that an advantage of DECT derived BMD analysis is 3D visualization of BMD distribution. For this, qCT would be an alternative scanning technology, but qCT scanners are less common, expose the patient to a higher radiation dose and require cross-manufacturer-calibration using suitable phantoms. Since a calibration phantom is necessary for every qCT scan, retrospective analysis of BMD cannot be performed.

An increasing number of CT examinations are performed with DECT due to the various possible applications in abdominal, cardiac, musculoskeletal, and vascular imaging. Patients and physicians would benefit from a technique that allows BMD assessment in all diagnostic DECT examinations virtually as a byproduct and that does not require phantom calibration or additional scan series. Automated BMD assessment when performing CT scans would also improve the hospital work flow and reduce medical costs.

A strong correlation between DECT and DXA could not be found. The main reason for this is the fact that DXA is a 2D projection technique. Thus, DXA images of vertebrae represent a mixture of cortical and trabecular bone absorption values. Given the fact that the cortical bone is able to compensate to some extent a lowered BMD of the trabecular bone, DXA is not sensitive enough for predicting fracture risks [11]. For this, DECT has a clear advantage since it allows for a separate examination of the trabecular bone. In a previous publication [10], we have demonstrated the strong correlation between our DECT-based BMD computation and measured pull-out forces. Since these local force measurements cannot be conducted in vivo, an additional qCT scanning would be desirable. Unfortunately, this would result in additional radiation exposure for the patient and is consequently hardly feasible.

There are limitations to this study. As usual, the inclusion of more patients would represent a stronger foundation for a statistical analysis. But, since we focused on demonstrating that DECT-based assessment of BMD is feasible in a clinical setting, this study was limited to 25 patients using the same DSCT scanner. A multi-center approach with a larger patient group and implementation of DSCT from various vendors is required to reassess the practicability of this technique in the clinical routine. Second, correlation studies with additional indicators of bone stability are necessary to demonstrate the potential advantage of sub-segmental BMD distribution analysis using DECT over conventional DXA.

In conclusion, we demonstrated that in vivo DECT-based BMD assessment of the lumbar spine in a clinical setting is feasible. As an advantage over DXA, this technique allows for computation of 3D spatial BMD distribution and therefore evaluation of regional stability of the trabecular bone of all osseous anatomic regions. Our technique allows for prospective as well as retrospective analysis of DECT data and therefore might further reduce the number of performed imaging examinations per patient, decrease radiation exposure for the patient and reduce medical costs.

References

1. Adams, J.E.: Quantitative computed tomography. Eur. J. Radiol. **71**(3), 415–424 (2009)
2. Blake, G.M., Fogelman, I.: The clinical role of dual energy X-ray absorptiometry. Eur. J. Radiol. **71**(3), 406–414 (2009)
3. Engelke, K., Adams, J.E., Armbrecht, G., Augat, P., Bogado, C.E., Bouxsein, M.L., Felsenberg, D., Ito, M., Prevrhal, S., Hans, D.B., Lewiecki, E.M.: Clinical use of quantitative computed tomography and peripheral quantitative computed tomography in the management of osteoporosis in adults: the 2007 ISCD official positions. J. Clin. Densitometry **11**(1), 123–162 (2008)
4. Erdt, M., Kirschner, M., Wesarg, S.: Simultaneous segmentation and correspondence establishment for statistical shape models. In: Magnenat-Thalmann, N. (ed.) 3DPH 2009. LNCS, vol. 5903, pp. 25–35. Springer, Heidelberg (2009)
5. Flohr, T.G., McCollough, C.H., Bruder, H., Petersilka, M., Gruber, K., Süß, C., Grasruck, M., Stierstorfer, K., Krauss, B., Raupach, R., Primak, A.N., Küttner, A., Achenbach, S., Becker, C., Kopp, A., Ohnesorge, B.M.: First performance evaluation of a dual-source CT (DSCT) system. Eur. Radiol. **16**(2), 256–268 (2006)
6. Genant, H.K., Boyd, D.: Quantitative bone mineral analysis using dual energy computed tomography. Invest. Radiol. **12**(6), 545–551 (1977)
7. Nickoloff, E.L., Feldman, F., Atherton, J.V.: Bone mineral assessment: new dual-energy CT approach. Radiology **168**(1), 223–228 (1988)
8. Singer, A.: Osteoporosis diagnosis and screening. Clin. Cornerstone **8**(1), 9–18 (2006)

9. van Kuijk, C., Grashuis, J.L., Steenbeek, J.C., Schütte, H.E., Trouerbach, W.T.: Evaluation of postprocessing dual-energy methods in quantitative computed tomography. Part 2. Practical aspects. Invest. Radiol. **25**(8), 882–889 (1990)

10. Wesarg, S., Kirschner, M., Becker, M., Erdt, M., Kafchitsas, K., Khan, M.F.: Dualenergy CT-based assessment of the trabecular bone in vertebrae. Meth. Inf. Med. **51**(5), 398–405 (2012)

11. WHO - World Health Organization: WHO Scientific Group on the Assessment of Osteoporosis at Primary Health Care Level (2007), summary Meeting Report Brussels, Belgium, 5–7 May 2004

12. Yoganandan, N., Pintar, F.A., Stemper, B.D., Baisden, J.L., Aktay, R., Shender, B.S., Paskoff, G., Laud, P.: Trabecular bone density of male human cervical and lumbar vertebrae. Bone **39**(2), 336–344 (2006)

Author Index